NEGOTIATING DEATH IN CONTEMPORARY HEALTH AND SOCIAL CARE

Margaret Holloway

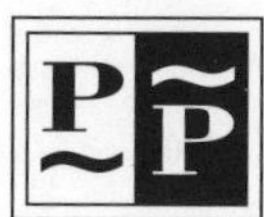

First published in Great Britain in 2007 by

The Policy Press
University of Bristol
Fourth Floor
Beacon House
Queen's Road
Bristol BS8 1QU
UK

Tel +44 (0)117 331 4054
Fax +44 (0)117 331 4093
e-mail tpp-info@bristol.ac.uk
www.policypress.org.uk

British Library Cataloguing in Publication Data
A catalogue record for this book is available from the British Library.

Library of Congress Cataloging-in-Publication Data
A catalog record for this book has been requested.

ISBN 978 1 86134 722 0 paperback
ISBN 978 1 84742 015 2 hardcover

Cover design by Qube Design Associates, Bristol
Front cover: photograph supplied by kind permission of Simon Cataudo.
Printed and bound in Great Britain by Hobbs the Printers, Southampton.

The Laughing Buddha

Beside the pond in our garden is a statuette of a laughing Buddha. He stands with arms stretched upwards in joyous celebration. Except that one arm is broken, the missing piece resting on the ground next to his feet. When the accident happened, I asked my husband to stick the piece back on. Noticing that the repair went undone for some considerable period of time, I enquired as to whether there was a problem. 'I quite like it like that', was the response. Over time I have come to agree with him. The wounded laughing Buddha speaks of joy reaching through pain, of severed connections nevertheless sustained. It has more to say than the perfect model.

Contents

List of tables and figures

Tables

Figures

Acknowledgements

Many people are owed my deepest thanks for their help and support. But for the insistence of the late Jo Campling this book might never have been written. Sue Adamson, Ben Fell and Jeanette Gilchrist undertook the comprehensive literature searches which provide the foundation for Chapters Five, Six and Seven. Sue Adamson is owed especial gratitude for compiling the mortality statistics contained in Chapters One and Six. John Creasey, Janet Dean, Anne English, Maureen George, Jo Gillespie, Ruth Hunter, Elaine Longley, Tracey Oliver, Wendy Price, Petra Van der Zand, Jill Walmsley and Ben Zylic generously provided me with a rich source of up-to-date case material and shared their professional selves with great honesty. Thanks are also due to Judith Hodgson for her endless enthusiasm for the project. My colleagues at the University of Hull generously allowed me time, and last but by no means least, my family have been endlessly patient with my pleas to be left alone! If I have done justice to them all, I am glad. If faults remain, they are mine alone.

ONE

Death in late modernity

Introduction

If there has to be a reason for another book on death, dying and bereavement, it is this: a subject which is of timeless significance for human beings as individuals, nevertheless is experienced in a social context, and that context is changing rapidly, irreversibly and, some would argue, fundamentally. Health and social care practitioners are both affected by these changes on a personal level and as professionals must negotiate their role and task to take account of this changing scene. It may be true that death is a universal human experience and in this sense the great leveller, but in every other respect it seems that dying and bereavement throw up a complex mesh of issues unique to the individual, yet shaped by prevailing social, political, legal, economic, philosophical, religious and cultural imperatives. The overarching theme of this book is that process of negotiation; its quest is the search for a knowledge base which is relevant and a practice framework which is 'fit for purpose' in contemporary health and social care settings. There is one principal limitation concerning the scope of the book which must be acknowledged at the outset. Neither global context nor cultural variation can be covered exhaustively although both are key themes in the argument and international examples and multicultural references are woven throughout. There is admittedly something of a focus on the UK but it is to be hoped that this serves to provide an in-depth starting point rather than exclusive discussion.

In this process of 'negotiating death' it is the context of the twenty-first century which determines the prevailing attitudes to death, the practices created to mark its occurrence and the accommodation of the experiences of dying and bereavement. There are individual, societal and specific community dimensions to that context, each of which makes its own very particular contribution to what may be termed the 'management' of death and dying. The individual makes his or her unique response on an emotional, psychological and spiritual level. This response is shaped and mediated by the society in which the individual is located, with its cultural, religious and behavioural norms – all of which tend to be remarkably prescribed where death is concerned. These social norms tend to be conveyed and impinge upon the individual through the response of their immediate community – although the relative influence of society and community in different environments is one of the issues with which we are concerned. As individuals we variously reflect such influences. As practitioners, we need to understand them with a breadth and depth which far extends our personal perspective. This complex context influences what practitioners feel able to talk about, and how, requiring sensitivity to a wide range of cultural perspectives and practices and the knowledge and skill to address them. It determines the response which they and their service organisation are able to make. The Australian government, for example, ordered a high-profile response through its own social work agency to the very public and traumatic disaster of Bali, where action taken by the UK government was deemed to be too little too late and not involving counselling agencies at all. Throughout this book we shall be exploring the knowledge base which will help us to engage with this context.

Postmodernism

In order to grapple with such a vast and challenging terrain, four factors will be considered which, arguably, are the principal shapers of contemporary death: *the predominant causes and patterns of death*; *the globalisation of death*; *shifting boundaries between public and private domains*; and, finally, *cultural pluralism*. As these headings suggest, they are each in their own way concerned with change, and they each cut across traditional academic boundaries to appear as connecting themes. These 'interconnecting conversations', or *discourses*, are a feature of a phenomenon which has come to be known as *postmodernism*. In this book we shall characterise the contemporary period as 'late modernity' because while the features of contemporary death have emerged out of modern societies, the picture being one of gradual shift which establishes a new order, but is still, in many ways, connected to the old. In order to better understand this process, however, it is helpful to look first at what is meant by postmodernism and its relevance to the study of death.

Christopher Butler, in his 'Very Short Introduction' to *Postmodernism*, characterises the intellectual stream of the movement as an 'excessively critical self-consciousness' (Butler, 2002, p. 6), which eschews overarching theory, claiming that all interpretations are partial and belong to the 'actor' who appropriates them. From this starting point, it is not surprising that postmodernist thought becomes preoccupied with themes of individual autonomy, of self and identity, of diversity and moral relativity, its hallmark being ontological uncertainty. Postmodernism is also a social movement, however, whose players are connected by the desire to resist narratives which have worked to bolster the power of a dominant group and oppress others; the most widely recognised example of this is the construction of patriarchal society which works according to rules and definitions laid down by men to preserve their power and interests over women. There is thus a socially created self which may, however, be at odds with the individually experienced self. Personal identity is arrived at through the interaction of both. In fact, recent work on identity emphasises the notion of identity as *process*, reached through a constant negotiation between the social structuring of self and the operation of individual agency (Jenkins, 2004).

How is this discussion relevant to contemporary death, dying and bereavement? First, and very simply, because it reminds us of the diversity of human experience in the face of a universal and irrefutable phenomenon. Postmodernist thinking also leads to the conclusion that the individual will make of their own death what they will. Small suggests that critical features of postmodernity for death are not simply consumerism, choice and difference, but the incorporation of reflexivity and irony, which 'challenges not just established procedures but also the status of the significant' (Small, 1997, p 205). This is particularly apt when we consider the attempts of professional helpers to guide dying and bereaved people through the best ways to die and to grieve and the laying down of prescribed care 'pathways' as 'best practice'. Gradually, we are learning more about the expert wisdom of the service user.

Another relevant theme is ontological uncertainty. Both Giddens and Craib are interested in ontological uncertainty in the face of death. Giddens suggests that in contemporary society we try to purchase ontological security through procedures and institutions which protect us from direct encounters with the reminders of those fundamental facts of existence which otherwise threaten us, such as madness and death. We try to find reliability in persons and things in order to shore up our sense of ourselves (Giddens, 1991). For Craib, however, the 'fragmented self' is a condition of contemporary society and the 'disappointed self', one which knows it does not have ultimate control, the only authentic position to surface in the face of death (Craib, 1994). Contemporary bereavement research is very much concerned with what happens when the narrative or script for my life or yours is disrupted or replaced.

Positions of moral relativity may at first sight seem to capture the ethics of end-of-life decision making and care but in fact here we find moral absolutes bumping into each other, particularly for the doctor whose duty is both to relieve suffering and to sustain life. Moreover, such positions are dictated by religious and cultural imperatives which may brook no negotiation of the relationship between human agency and the boundary of life and death. Nevertheless, we find such negotiation of necessity going on in the context of pluralist societies.

The importance of culture in postmodern theorising cannot be overstated. Culture as a concept has the capacity to embrace sociological, philosophical and psychological perspectives, allowing it to emerge from the static descriptions used to characterise societies in the second half of the twentieth century. Culture has come to denote a more dynamic interplay between concepts of identity and meaning, policy themes, organisational constructs and organised practices. It is thus a crucial concept when we come to look at death, dying and bereavement. Cultural pluralism also generates plural identities for the individual. Both feminism and disability politics have rediscovered that the individual may experience several identities simultaneously and these are not necessarily hierarchically ordered. They may, however, be situation-dependent. 'Who am I?' is a question which the dying or bereaved person may find hard to answer, and sometimes begs the question 'Who are you?' before communication can be established. Questions of individual and social identity are crucial to the way in which death is approached and managed, whether the role is as a dying or bereaved person, a helping person or professional, or an affected community.

Finally, what does postmodern theorising contribute to our theorising of death, dying and bereavement? An understanding of death which is embedded in context but does not seek overarching explanation seems an appropriate quest for the better understanding of contemporary dying and bereavement. At the same time, we are constantly brought back to death's fundamental and universal relationship with human existence; Beckford, in his critique of postmodernist thought on religion and society, reminds us of the importance of anchor points if we are to better understand and progress (Beckford, 1996). Butler (2002) concludes that postmodernism has provided a useful and timely critique but it does not supersede all other intellectual traditions.

Causes and patterns of death

One of the most important determiners of the way in which death is managed in any society is its demographic profile: who is dying, at what ages, from what causes, in what physical and social circumstances? The literature on which health and social care professionals may draw to begin to understand the experiences of dying and bereavement has been built up from research and clinical practice which has largely focused on death in two categories: first, death from terminal illness, which has tended to mean cancer; and second, deaths which are in some way 'special', predominantly a range of 'sudden deaths' such as suicide, in public disasters (although disaster theory developed more recently in the 1980s), or untimely deaths, such as the death of a child. Whilst these categorisations continue to have relevance, they provide us with only a partial picture of death in the early twenty-first century. Moreover, examination of the causes and patterns of death, looking at current figures, trends and forecasted mortality rates, suggests that the majority dying is shifting, particularly in developed countries.

The pattern now emerging relates to the phenomenon of population ageing. Although it is common to refer to an ageing population, there are a number of variations on this trend, which are significant when it comes to the picture of death in any one society at a given time. The 'problem' of an aged dependent population was first noted in northern and western Europe, where we see slow ageing of an already aged population, produced through a combination of static birth rates and slowly falling death rates. This pattern also applies to America, Canada and Australia but here it is combined with markedly higher death rates among younger immigrant populations. Japan, China and Latin America, meanwhile, are experiencing very rapid ageing, resulting from low birth rates alongside falling death rates. In most parts of the developing world, by comparison, we see relatively slow ageing, where in a previously young population, death rates are falling faster than birth rates, which, however, are also falling. Finally, in Eastern Europe and the former USSR, low birth rates and static death rates combine to produce slow ageing but from an intermediate position (Wilson, 2000). Overall, the World Health Organization predicts that average life expectancy worldwide will be 75 years by 2025, with no country less than 50 years, but this in fact tells us very little about the experiences of dying or bereavement in any one country. So, for example, the homicide rate in Russia had climbed to the highest in the world by 1993–4 (Seale, 2000) and the AIDS pandemic has significantly set back parts of Africa, as well as creating a generation which is both orphaned and HIV positive. Meanwhile, the UK and US are preoccupied with large numbers dying in very old age from, or with, chronic diseases – the Institute of Medicine quotes 2.4 million Americans dying in old age each year (IOM, 2003). Despite this majority pattern of dying, the UK has some startling pockets of social and health inequalities, which makes sobering reading for a developed country in the twenty-first century.

Death in the UK

The 2004 death rate for all ages in the UK was 9.5 per 1000 population for males and 10.0 per 1000 population for females. There are more male deaths in all age groups except those aged 85 and over where there are more than twice as many female deaths. There is a general increase in death rates and numbers of deaths with age, and higher rates per 1000 population at all ages in males than in females.

Figure 1.1: Death rates in the UK 2004, by age and gender

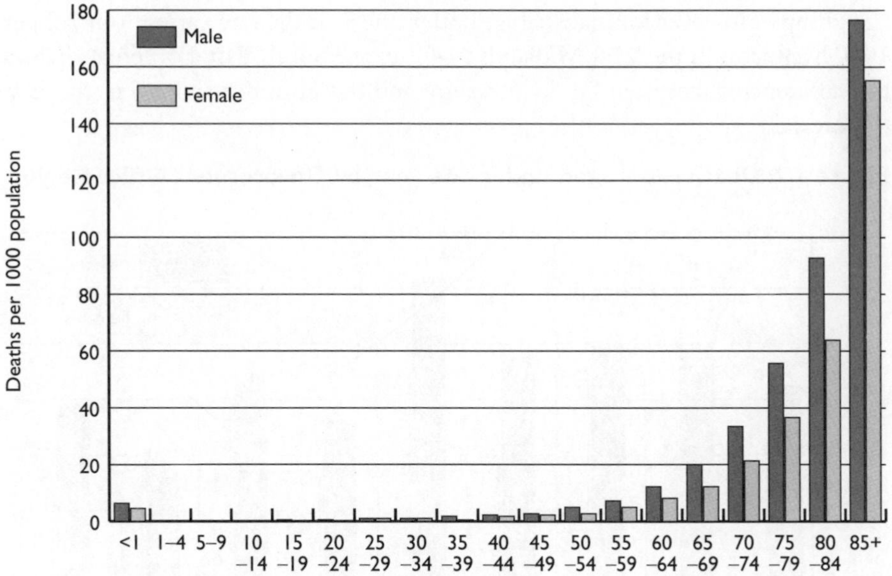

Source: Series DH1 no 37 Mortality Statistics ONS 2006

Death rates for deaths at all ages vary across the country as shown in Table 1.1. London has the lowest rates and Scotland the highest rates for both males and females.

Table 1.1: Variations across the UK

	Males	Females
	Rate per 1000 population	
England	9.3	9.8
Wales	10.6	11.1
Scotland	10.9	11.2
Northern Ireland	8.3	8.5
Government Office Regions		
North East	10.7	11.0
North West	10.2	10.7
Yorkshire and the Humber	9.8	10.3
East Midlands	9.5	10.0
West Midlands	9.7	10.0
East	9.2	9.8
London	7.1	7.4
South East	9.0	9.9
South West	10.1	10.8

Source: Series DH1 no 37 Mortality Statistics ONS 2006

Within England and Wales there generally is little variation in death rates between the Government Office Regions for children, young and middle-aged age groups. However for male babies under one year the rate varies from 7.2 per 1000 live births in the West Midlands to 4.1 in the South East. For female babies the difference is between 5.5 in Yorkshire and the Humber and 3.7 in the East (Figure 1.2).

Figure 1.2: Death rates aged under one year, by Government Office Region

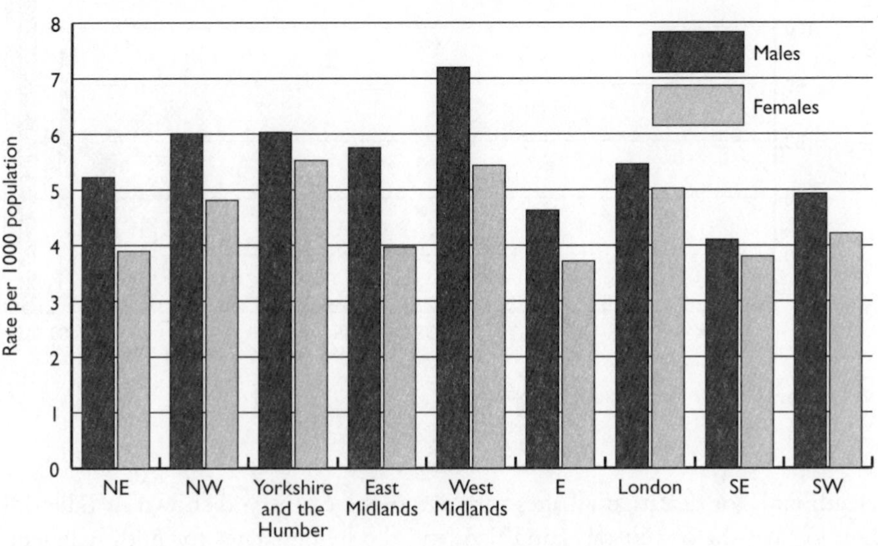

Source: Series DH1 no 37 Mortality Statistics ONS 2006

There is also variation in older age groups, the same pattern appearing of higher rates in the north and lower rates in the south for both males and females in the three age groups (Figure 1.3).

Figure 1.3: Death rates at older ages, by Government Office Region

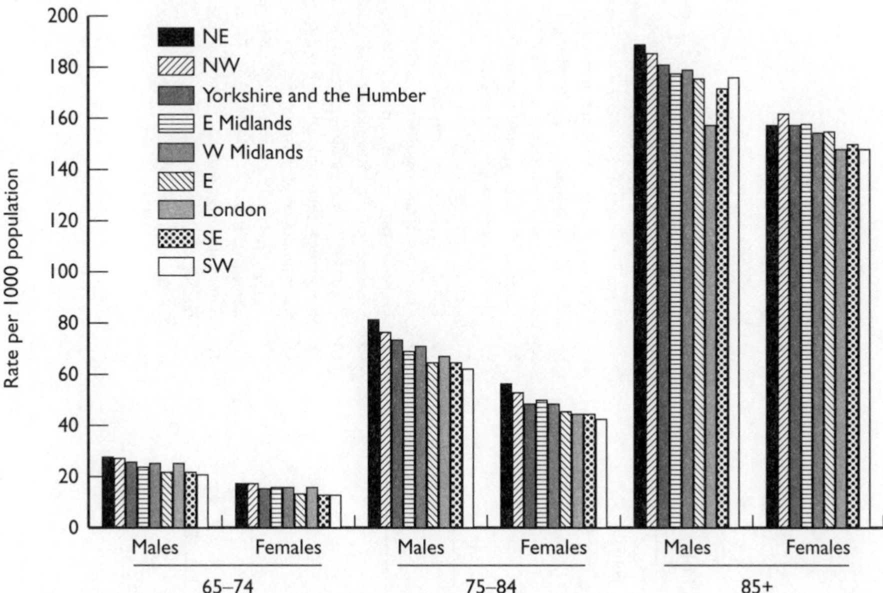

Source: Series DH1 no 37 Mortality Statistics ONS 2006

Causes of death

The main causes of death for all ages are diseases of the circulatory system, neoplasms and, to a lesser extent, diseases of the respiratory system (Figure 1.4).

The major causes of death overall identified an increase in rates per million population with age, being relatively low in younger people but increasing sharply in middle age (Figures 1.5 and 1.6). For example, cancers account for only 30 deaths per million or fewer in younger people but in the oldest males reach over 30,000 per million. Circulatory diseases have the highest rates for oldest age groups but cancer has higher rates at ages up to 74. Digestive diseases have higher rates than respiratory diseases in those aged 25–44 but for other age groups the position is reversed. Male deaths from circulatory diseases increase particularly sharply at age 35–44, while for females in that age range the rise is most substantial in cancer. In the older age groups cancer is more prevalent for males than females but in middle age the reverse is true.

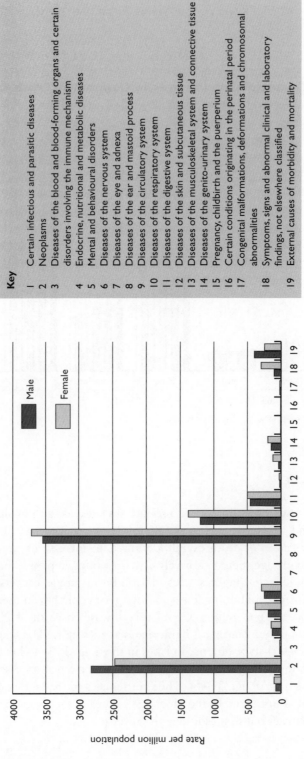

Figure 1.4: Cause of death in the UK by gender

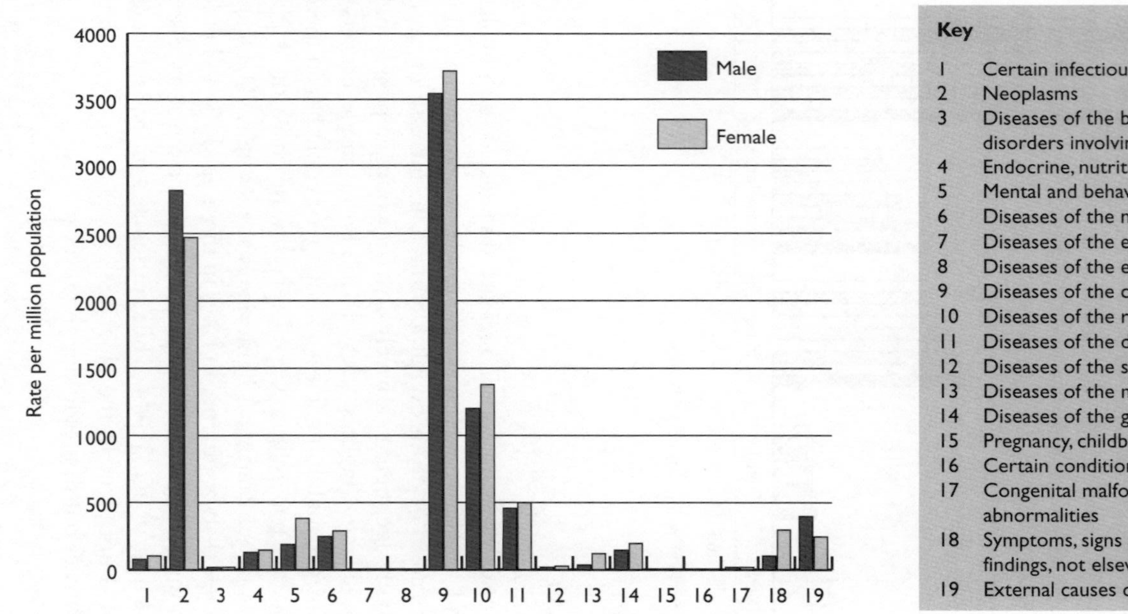

Key

1 Certain infectious and parasitic diseases
2 Neoplasms
3 Diseases of the blood and blood-forming organs and certain disorders involving the immune mechanism
4 Endocrine, nutritional and metabolic diseases
5 Mental and behavioural disorders
6 Diseases of the nervous system
7 Diseases of the eye and adnexa
8 Diseases of the ear and mastoid process
9 Diseases of the circulatory system
10 Diseases of the respiratory system
11 Diseases of the digestive system
12 Diseases of the skin and subcutaneous tissue
13 Diseases of the musculoskeletal system and connective tissue
14 Diseases of the genito-urinary system
15 Pregnancy, childbirth and the puerperium
16 Certain conditions originating in the perinatal period
17 Congenital malformations, deformations and chromosomal abnormalities
18 Symptoms, signs and abnormal clinical and laboratory findings, not elsewhere classified
19 External causes of morbidity and mortality

Source: Series DH1 no 37 Mortality Statistics ONS 2006

Figure 1.5: Major causes of death in younger people 2004

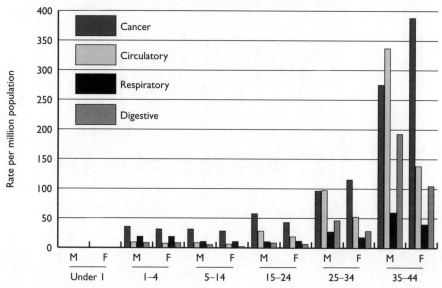

Source: Series DH1 no 37 Mortality Statistics ONS 2006

Figure 1.6: Major causes of death in older age groups 2004

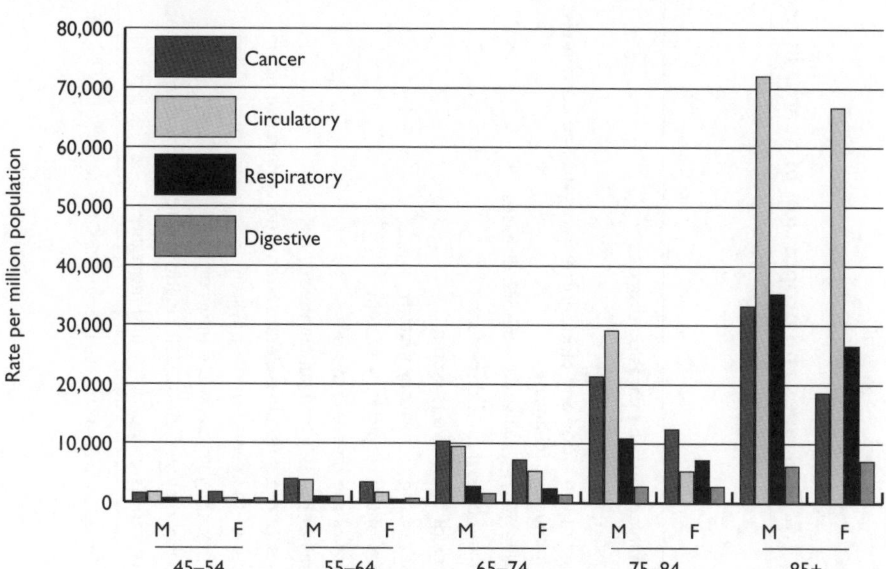

Source: Series DH1 no 37 Mortality Statistics ONS 2006

Table 1.2: Peak ages and proportion of deaths in age group

	Male		Female	
	Peak age	Percentage	Peak age	Percentage
Certain infectious and parasitic diseases	1–4	8.71	1–4	10.92
Neoplasms	60–64	41.25	55–59	55.53
Diseases of the blood and blood-forming organs and certain disorders involving the immune mechanism	1–4	2.09	5–9	3.01
Endocrine, nutritional and metabolic diseases	5–9	7.65	1–4	8.73
Mental and behavioural disorders	25–29	9.25	90–94	6.27
Diseases of the nervous system	1–4	17.07	5–9	14.29
Diseases of the circulatory system	85–89	41.8	85–89	44.52
Diseases of the respiratory system	95 and over	24.5	95 and over	20.55
Diseases of the digestive system	45–49	13.13	40–44	10.61
Diseases of the skin and subcutaneous tissue	95 and over	0.31	95 and over	0.55
Diseases of the musculoskeletal system and connective tissue	90–94	0.89	10–14	2.45
Diseases of the genito-urinary system	95 and over	3.71	95 and over	2.91
Pregnancy, childbirth and the puerperium			30–34	1.98
Congenital malformations, deformations and chromosomal abnormalities	1–4	12.89	1–4	13.54
External causes of morbidity and mortality	15–19	62.58	15–19	42.93

Source: Series DH2 no 37 Mortality Statistics ONS 2006

Place of death

By far the largest numbers of deaths take place in NHS hospitals, as shown in Figure 1.7. Rather more female than male deaths take place in hospitals other than NHS, and in other communal establishments, and more male than female at home or in other private houses.

Figure 1.7: Place of death 2004

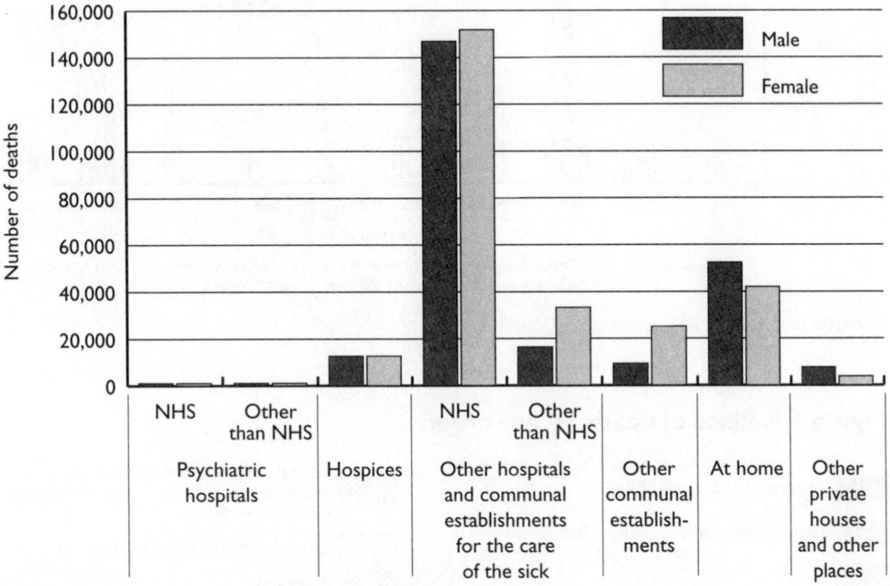

Number of deaths
160,000
140,000
120,000
100,000
80,000
60,000
40,000
20,000
0
Male
Female
NHS
Other than NHS
Psychiatric hospitals
Hospices
NHS
Other than NHS
Other hospitals and communal establishments for the care of the sick
Other communal establish-ments
At home
Other private houses and other places

Source: Series DH1 no 37 Mortality Statistics ONS 2006

For the main places of death there are some differences in numbers of deaths by age and gender (Figure 1.8). In NHS hospitals there are similar numbers of deaths at age 75–84 but more female deaths at age 85 and over. The larger numbers of female deaths in 'other than NHS hospitals and other than communal establishments' is the result of the disproportionate number of female deaths at this age. There are more male deaths in middle age in NHS hospitals and more male deaths at age 75–84 at home.

The proportion of deaths in different locations varies by age group (Figure 1.9). A larger proportion of the very young and the elderly than teenagers and middle-aged people die in NHS hospitals. These groups are more likely to die at home or in hospices. Only the very elderly are likely to die in communal establishments other than those for the care of the sick – presumably in homes for the elderly. There is little difference in these patterns by gender.

This picture of death and dying is extremely significant for health and social care practice. If most people now die in old age, from one of the diseases of old age, and usually in the hospital where they have recently been admitted from either their

Figure 1.8: Main places of death, by age group and gender

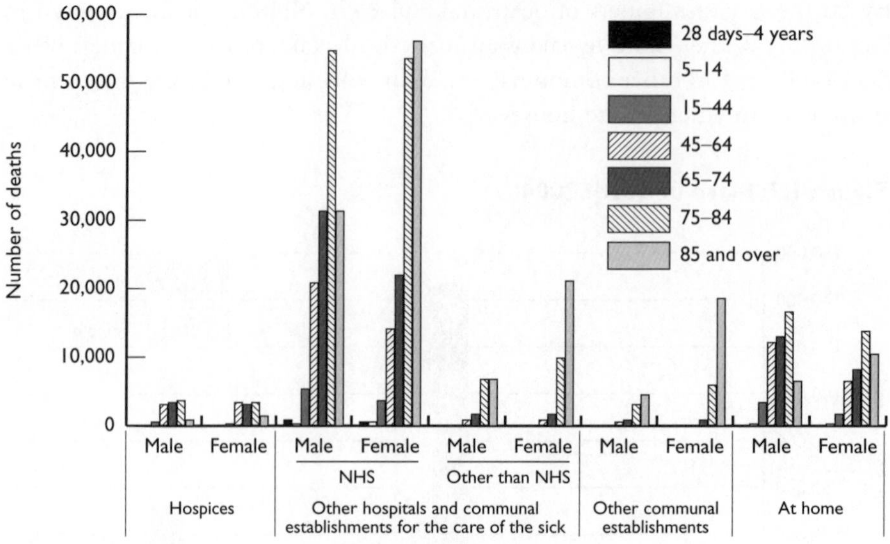

Source: Series DH1 no 37 Mortality Statistics ONS 2006

Figure 1.9: Place of death, by age group

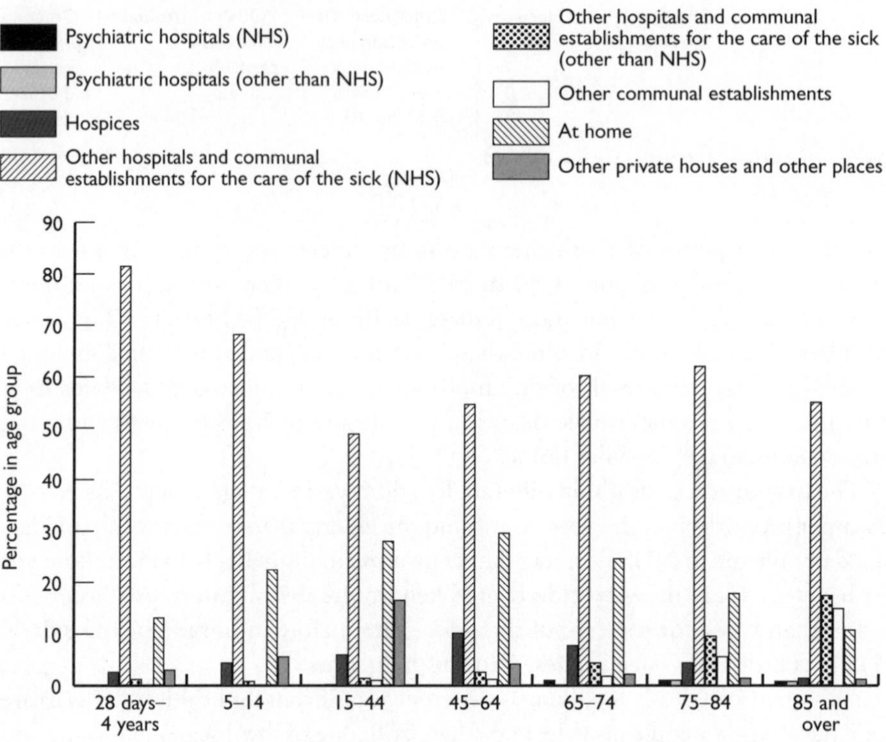

Source: Series DH1 no 37 Mortality Statistics ONS 2006

own home or a care home, it may be that the types of dying around which we have built our practice are not those that we increasingly find ourselves encountering. The challenge may be to transfer the good practice developed in palliative and hospice care to address the needs of 'mainstream' contemporary dying. Similarly, if types of deaths are emerging as a significant and hitherto unremarked 'minority dying', carrying with them the features usually attributed to 'special deaths', our knowledge base may need considerable and rapid expansion if we are to respond sensitively and appropriately to the needs of people so bereaved. Our value systems may be challenged by questions of who merits what treatment and for how long. Our empathy may be stretched as grief which was hitherto ignored or death previously seen only on a distant stage is brought close to home.

Globalisation of death

One of the features of globalisation which is particularly significant for our response as individuals and societies to death and dying is that images of death, and the responses of the societies in which they occur, are communicated across the world. This has a curious impact, creating both immediacy and distance. Those deaths are of two types. The first is the shocking face of unnatural or multiple deaths – sometimes on a massive scale – that are commonly a result of war, famine, natural disaster and human-induced tragic, sometimes horrific, events. The most recent example of such a disaster is the Asian tsunami that occurred on 26 December 2004. Its impact was not only immediate, as scenes of devastation appeared on television screens worldwide, but has continued, because global travel resulted in westerners being caught up in the tragedy. The destruction of the New York World Trade Center in a terrorist attack unfolded its horrors in front of us all, and has gone on to create the phenomenon known as '9/11', representative of a widely experienced threat which some have termed existential. The second type of image involves the reporting of the individual deaths of high-profile figures, or individual deaths which become high profile because of their circumstances, such as the Soham murders in which the public hunt first for the bodies and then for the murderer of two 10-year-old girls, fixated the British public. Sometimes the deaths of celebrity figures also illustrate areas of rising concern – such as Ronald Reagan suffering from dementia, Rock Hudson dying of AIDS and Pope John Paul II's physical decline as he was increasingly affected by both Parkinson's disease and ageing.

On the one hand it can be argued that these deaths are so far removed from the living rooms of most viewers that the phenomenon serves to further persuade us that death is 'out there' and need not concern us, until we are confronted with our own dying or the death of someone close. Exley argues that this results in a familiarity with death but with 'no investment of emotional capital' (Exley, 2004, p 111). I am inclined to think that this may not be the case. The helplines advertised after TV programmes dealing with difficult issues around death and dying for anyone 'affected by anything in this programme' indicate that the experience of programme makers is that people appropriate the emotions to themselves. The reaction of ordinary members of the public in the UK to the death of Diana, Princess of Wales, suggested a considerable emotional investment from large numbers of people, which commentators have variously speculated had to do with the opportunity to explore their own private griefs. Watson traces how this process, orchestrated through the media, resulted in Diana being raised to sainthood as the 'royal sacrificial victim' (Watson, 1997, p 6). A slightly different phenomenon may be occurring in relation to the deaths of ordinary citizens in extraordinary circumstances which are broadcast through the world media – soldiers and civilians in conflict zones or hostage victims, for example. The manner in which the stories of each casualty are told by the media, conveying family circumstances and featuring pleas and responses from family members, fosters an identification with those personal stories so that they seem to be as the deaths of everyone's child or parent.

The impact of these global images in confronting individuals with, and raising common awareness of, death and dying is, arguably, a significant factor in bringing death once more 'into the midst of life', where earlier sociologies of death and dying had demonstrated that it was shunted away. What it also does is to emphasise the commonality of human experiences and emotions in contexts in which the customs and rituals surrounding death may be quite different. This has the potential to serve as an important corrective to preconceived notions about the management of death and dying in situations alien to one's own. Life is not cheap just because people are dying in their thousands, and the grief of a parent when yet another child dies of dysentery is palpable for the TV viewer on the other side of the world. It also, however, demonstrates very sharply differences in belief. For example, after the tsunami, the burning of bodies of westerners by Buddhist monks before they could be identified and returned to their relatives, provoked profound disquiet and emphasised how significant, at individual and social levels, are beliefs about the body.

This form of opening up of death and dying can make a positive contribution to our approach as individuals and societies to death and dying, and it can also have a negative impact. Practitioners need to be alert to both possibilities. On the positive side, we should all be better placed to understand some of the complexities of difference at the same time as we are able to recognise the connections of common meaning which exist in our pluralist communities. Our own ignorance and unconscious prejudice as professionals may be lessened if not removed. Particular high-profile events may provide the opening to address topics on which the direct approach might prove too threatening to the service user. In a research project in which Chinese older people were encouraged to talk about their attitudes to cancer, the cancer and eventual death of a popular Chinese singer that had been closely followed in the media proved a useful trigger for the focus groups (Payne et al, 2005). There is, however, a downside to the widespread portrayals of death through media which are also used for entertainment and fantasy. It is possible that people may become used to treating death as outside of themselves and their experience, inured to images which, if they considered fully their meaning, might lead to feelings that they do not wish to confront. There is also the negative impact of conveying not only the image but also a social context which carries with it a stigmatising moral message. The death of a popular idol from a drug overdose, for example, has the potential to fuel all those local stories of heroin-using teenagers. The loneliness and stigma experienced by bereaved families in these situations is acute, and their treatment by health and social care professionals sometimes less than sympathetic (Guy and Holloway, 2007).

Shifting boundaries between the public and the private

Warren Smith comments that boundaries are a feature of the modern world (Smith, 2006). We are familiar with the way these are created and reinforced in public discourse, policy-making and social organisations. However, it is in our behaviours and interactions that we negotiate and renegotiate boundaries. A feature of late modernity is that boundaries once thought immutable are seen to be shifting and permeable. Death itself is no longer the clear-cut physical boundary which once it was and it is mediated through a number of other social features. One of these which impacts particularly on society's view of death and its individual experiences of dying and bereavement concerns what is deemed to belong to the public domain and what is deemed to be private. Late modernity has seen a dramatic shift in the boundary between the public and the private. The explosion in 'reality TV' and its undoubted widespread popularity and obsessive qualities (whilst also being repeatedly decried) is one universally recognisable example that appears to have global resonance.

Elizabeth Frazer (2000) argues that the distinction between 'public' and 'private' is drawn in four significant ways in the arenas of legal, political and social life. First, a distinction is made between private and public actions; second, between private and public worlds; third, between private and public interests; and, fourth, between private and public persona. These distinctions are helpful in trying to understand how death, as both a public and a private event, is changing in our society, particularly for professionals trying to negotiate those shifting boundaries.

Funerals

One of the key facets of contemporary death in which we see the boundaries shifting between what is publicly regulated and shared and what is deemed a private matter is in the events and procedures which follow immediately after a death, at the heart of which is the funeral. Since the 1960s it has been commonplace to assert that contemporary western society is stripped of social customs and rituals to steer its way through death, our ceremonies brief and meaningless, mourning socially acceptable only in the immediate period after the death and our grief kept private. Elias (1985) describes this as the 'loneliness' which attends both dying and grieving. Wouters attributes the decline in social rituals around death which were seen in the mid-twentieth century to a shift in the 'We–I' balance (Elias, 1991) which occurred in the pursuit of individualism (Wouters, 2002). However, Wouters goes on to suggest that the 1980s – a period in the UK in which individualism was at its height – saw the beginnings of the quest for new rituals to mark death. A decade or so on, Hockey argues that there is evidence of a rich and complex diversity of practice around death, but it is less routinised and more individually customised than previously, and thus not recognised as ritual (Hockey, 2001).

In fact, the trend to personalise funeral, mortuary and burial or other disposal practices has grown apace, and is increasingly public. These 'private touches' are shared. As Frazer so accurately observes: 'There is a kind of "privacy" which seems to draw its meaning only from being publicised' (Frazer, 2000, p 214). So a wider community of mourners comes to know aspects of the person which before were known only to the family; the family see a side to their relative recognised before only by colleagues. The inscription on the grave proclaims forever the essence of the person as remembered by those closest to them. The floral tributes displayed at the roadside are deeply intimate. It is not so much that we have substituted private shut-away behaviours for social rituals, as that personal feelings and behaviours are becoming the new public rituals, all the while imbued with private symbolic meaning. At the heart of this, Grainger argues that the funeral has become a way of establishing combined private and public meaning, rather than a way of behaving which represents socially prescribed meaning (Grainger, 1998). Gardner, reporting a study of funeral and burial practices among Bengali Muslims in Tower Hamlets, East London, suggests that practices which were formerly private are being brought into the public domain. In some instances, widows are breaking with tradition and attending the funeral (Gardner, 1998).

As with any significant change, and particularly one which cuts deep into some of our most fundamental social and psychological processes, this redefining of 'public' and 'private' in the arena of death and dying is not taking place without confusion and alarm. The immediate aftermath of the death of Diana, Princess of Wales, provides one of the clearest illustrations of some of these confusions, compounded by the tricky position of a popular public figure who had lost her constitutional public status, and whose own style was to bring personal and intimate touches into the public event, not stopping short of making the private confessional a public occasion. Frazer (2000) analyses how the British press tied itself up in knots as it commented on the Royal Family's initial protestations of protecting the grieving princes, only to ultimately sanction the adorning of the cortège with a floral tribute spelling 'MUMMY'; of the announcement that the funeral was neither state nor public, but a private funeral staged as a public event; of the constitutional position where the next of kin are both the monarchic line and 'first family' but the deceased is a private citizen; of the ownership of grief and whether the Royal Family should share the grief of the people.

Table 1.3: Merging of the public and the private in funerals

Public and private	Funerals
Actions	Personal touches in social ceremony
Worlds	Private life on public stage
Interests	Individual concerns juxtaposed with prescribed group behaviours
Persona	Intimate relationship becomes chief mourner

Home as the site of professional care

One of the objectives of health and social care policy in the western world, which has become more prominent since the 1990s, is to keep people who need care in their own homes for as long as possible. This has extended way beyond the range of standard domiciliary services to include quite sophisticated medical treatments, particularly in the field of cancer treatments and palliative care. People undergoing chemotherapy, with the apparatus attached, are encouraged, if they feel well enough, to go to work. 'Hospice-at-home' initiatives are among the fastest growing across Europe, North America and Australasia. Increasingly, admissions to a hospice or hospital take place only in the last few days of life. The oldest old, who may be both frail and suffering from one or more serious health conditions, are kept going through a battery of professional interventions usually in conjunction with high levels of care provided by family members, who may themselves be 'trained up' to administer treatments at one time regarded as requiring professional skills. Most significantly, the more this fusion of private circumstance and professional care can be achieved, the more it is regarded as 'best practice'. However, this effectively results in 'home' being turned into a place populated by strangers, where family assume unfamiliar roles and technology replaces homeliness.

Some have suggested that this blurring of boundaries is changing the character of 'home' so that it is questionable whether it still retains its comforting essence (Milligan, 2000; Brown, 2003). In the same vein, it is pointed out that 'home' may involve deprivations and be devoid of the components of individual love and care and loved ones which constitute the ideal of the 'warm hearth' (Gott et al, 2004). The objectives of good institutional care are now framed around personal and homely touches, and supported living complexes attempt to meld public and private spaces, although communal lounges may be rarely used and residents of individual flats may have only the warden's visits for company. Residents of care homes may be strongly encouraged to participate in communal activities and to sit in the day room, at the same time as staff are required to knock before entering private bedrooms. Moreover, the treatment of the sick or crumbling body occurs across public and private spaces, until such point as the individual's condition means that they can no longer be managed in public without discomforting others. Ethnographic accounts of hospital wards and nursing homes show how death becomes private, or sequestered, even within public care (Lawton, 2000), although Froggatt (2001) suggests the creation of transitional states between the living and the dying. The social abandonment experienced by many older people

Table 1.4: Public and private aspects of care

Public and private	Care
Actions	Home equipped like hospital; homely touches in institutional care
Worlds	Melding of public and private spaces in care settings; care/treatment of sick body in public places
Interests	Individual abandoned to public care; death sequestered in public institutions
Persona	Professional carers at home; relatives assume professional roles at home and in institutions

living alone in their own homes is mirrored in the experience of many in the communal home: 'Some had been abandoned by their next of kin and the days followed each other in silence and without conversation' (Franklin et al, 2006, p 139).

Cultural pluralism

The ways in which death is experienced and marked are at the heart of culture and religion. Indeed, Reimers (1999) analyses the funerals of three immigrant communities and a municipal cemetery in Sweden, to demonstrate that these rituals and symbols of death are of themselves a means of promoting cultural identity. When looking at death in late modernity, we are dealing with both cultural diversity and cross-cultural issues simultaneously. Although we are not short of social anthropological studies to increase our knowledge of the making and employing of death rituals within and across cultures (for example, Metcalfe and Huntington, 1991), the failure in the original theoretical modellings of dying and bereavement to accommodate social and cultural difference is recognised as a major deficit. This has particular impact on practitioners seeking to apply this knowledge to their work in multicultural contexts where pluralism of belief is a significant factor. One of the drivers in the development of the theory of continuing bonds, which at first sight is something of an overturning of previously established wisdom, has been the 'discovery' that maintaining bonds with those who have died appears to coexist quite easily with getting on with life in non-western cultures (Klass and Goss, 1999).

More recent work has begun to address cultural diversity by providing accounts of dying and bereavement in different cultures set alongside each other (for example, Irish, 1993; Parkes et al, 1996). On specific aspects, Clark and Seymour (1999) address the influence of different ontological assumptions on culturally prescribed patterns of dying and mourning, and Klass and Goss (1999) have explored the importance of spiritual bonds in Japanese and western cultures. In a fascinating collection of essays exploring the interweaving of death, gender and ethnicity, Field et al (1997) provide a largely sociological analysis (although Thompson, in his discussion of masculinity and loss, does refer to the importance of ontology). Deeken, out of his examination of changing rituals and beliefs in Japan, concludes that there are more commonalities than differences in the bereavement experience of people from different cultural backgrounds (Deeken, 2004). Meanwhile, Walter argues for distinctly different traditions even within western culture, suggesting that the process of secularisation and the relationship between religious and secular institutions have developed separately in the US, Britain and Europe; thus the way in which religious minorities adapt in each context will also be different (Walter, 2005).

In some instances, the cultural context causes a shift in the symbolic value of a practice. From mainstream western culture, Jean Seaton (2006) regrets the fact that black has become a fashion colour, stripping it of its symbolic value in mourning. Pollack reports from a study of survivors in Srebrenica that achieving proper burial in the homeland of those massacred by the Serbs became linked in the minds of survivors with their case for repatriation (Pollack, 2003). Similarly, work emerging from Israel suggests that tensions between the individual and personal and sociopolitical dynamics dominate the bereavement experiences of relatives of people killed in suicide bomber attacks, and this may well be transferable to other victims of terrorist attacks around the world (Ronel and Lebel, 2006). Dying at home for Hong Kong Chinese, both those remaining in Hong Kong and those who have settled in the UK, no longer represents the spirit at peace, since in both Hong Kong and the UK, houses change hands quite frequently. Thus, many older people express the desire for their remains to be taken back to the ancestral home in mainland China. As an alternative, the practice is developing in some UK cities of a ceremony to return the remains symbolically to the ancestral home (Payne et al, 2005). Both Jonker (1997) and Reimers (1999) concluded that for some migrant communities the funeral can be a 'funeral in exile', representing a mix of retaining and adapting original traditions to the adopted context – often out of practical necessity. Reimers goes on to conclude that the cultural identity promoted is not necessarily the ethnicity, citing the examples in Sweden of a Polish Mormon for whom being a Mormon was more important than being Polish, and a Catholic Polish woman whose funeral was a synthesis of Polish, Swedish and Christian traits.

Thus, cultural pluralism as expressed in death in late modernity is a complex tapestry of defined, tightly woven and faintly delineated threads. Gadberry (2000) comments that the process which facilitates social shifts is commonly a melding of old traditions and new practices which coexist for some considerable period before the shift occurs. This process may be comforting, confusing or alien for individuals. Important as the work to date is in progressing our overview understanding of death in contemporary society, we still lack the breadth and depth of empirical research which investigates subjective meaning for the individual, experienced within a particular cultural context. This is increasingly important in a world not simply of cultural diversity, but of individuals straddling cultures and traditions and experiencing major social transition. Gunaratnam is scathing in her attack on 'cultural reductionism' and 'cultural and religious prescription', leading to, 'a tendency to project and confuse private feelings with public behaviour ... [and] oversimplified assumptions about the relationships between ritual behaviour, social support and subjective grief' (1997, p. 177).

Conclusion

Death is both absent and present in contemporary society. There is continuing evidence that we push it away, sometimes shutting it out of sight by the very structures set up in health and social care to deal with dying. Yet contemporary dying is a process in which we intervene, control and manage – as individual citizens and professionals – as never before. Contemporary experiences of bereavement have characteristics which we are only just beginning to note and to understand. At the same time, other aspects have enduring relevance and we in the twenty-first century struggle with the same experiences of loss and suffering as human beings have always done. The context for our struggle, however, is in some respects fundamentally different from that of previous centuries and generations. This chapter has outlined key demographic, social and cultural features of that context. These themes will recur within the ensuing chapters. An important dynamic underlying the whole is its philosophical context. Death cannot but raise existential questions and the management of death, whether through social rituals and structures, religious and cultural systems or policy frameworks, raises important philosophical and ethical questions and reflects dominant positions.

This is a tricky terrain to traverse. Individuals must deal with death for themselves when it comes their way, but there are multitudes of health and social care professionals with whom they might come into contact in so doing. This is the case more now than ever before. These professionals may be more or less helpful or they may even hinder, depending on the relevance and depth of their knowledge and their ability to relate with sensitivity to the other person and their situation. This book is not a handbook for practice but it does attempt to critically appraise that knowledge base in the light of issues for practice. The remaining chapters examine the field of contemporary death, dying and bereavement from academic and practice perspectives, with the aim of providing an interdisciplinary and interprofessional encounter. It is a challenging agenda and inevitably there are omissions. My hope is that the map and the journey are sufficiently clear and thought-provoking to encourage the reader to continue alone.

TWO

Contemporary health and social care

Introduction

The social and demographic changes outlined in Chapter One have also created a situation in which dying has become the business of professional services. Very few people now live their lives to the end, in their own homes, without any recourse to formal health or social care services. For the vast majority of people dying in old age, these service providers will be involved to a greater or lesser extent with their lives, and the lives of their families, often intensively in the last few weeks or days. For the younger person who dies suddenly and unexpectedly, perhaps as a result of accident or injury, accident and emergency services will be called upon not only to deal with the medical emergency but also to support the bereaved relatives. Thus the ways in which health and social care services are organised and delivered have a profound effect on the experiences of dying and bereavement and also on the ways in which the individual professional may seek to offer help. These services have themselves been subject to considerable change and challenge in the late twentieth and early twenty-first centuries. In the developed societies of Europe and North America, the pace of national policy change has been rapid and can be seen to reflect common global trends as these societies respond to the overlapping health and social needs of an increasing sector of the population which requires more intensive interventions over a longer period of time (Tester, 1996; Walker and Maltby, 1997). In the developing world, the scale of epidemics, such as the HIV/AIDS crisis in Africa, has required the rapid training of non-professional healthcare workers who deal with death on a daily basis and in large numbers.

This chapter takes as its starting point the contemporary scene in the UK, which has an established theoretical and practical tradition in work with people who are dying and bereaved. The issues and developments highlighted, however, are paralleled in other parts of Europe, North America, Australasia and Hong Kong. The predominance of chronic illness and co-morbidities alongside continuously improving survivor rates for cancer have made the establishment of an integrated health and social care system, which is effective and equitable for all, a priority in the developed world. The problems of fragmented services at the point of delivery, health inequalities particularly experienced by immigrant and ethnic minority populations, and top-down, government and service-driven responses rather than bottom-up patient-centred care are common frustrations of that overarching aim. The US Institute of Medicine's aims for healthcare in the twenty-first century are that it should be patient-centred, effective, timely, efficient, equitable and safe

(IOM, 2001). These aims are echoed throughout the developed world. Its strategy for achieving these aims, with an emphasis on interdisciplinary working, evidence-based practice and a better educated, more flexible and diverse workforce, are similarly reflected in other national policy initiatives.

Before examining the broad context of health and social care services, let us consider the settings in which practitioners are working with dying and bereaved people. It is sometimes assumed that this is a specialist area of practice confined to hospices and some hospital teams. In fact, any practitioner working in the human services may encounter a person whose problems stem from, or are exacerbated by, grief or who is involved with someone who is dying. Care of the person who is dying from cancer or another acute condition is concentrated in hospices and specialist palliative care units within hospitals, but end-of-life care for the older person, or the person with a slowly degenerating condition, may be provided through primary care and general services. As specialist palliative care services are increasingly delivered in the home, routine community care services may contribute to the support of the dying person and their family. Accident and emergency services and the formal proceedings which sometimes follow sudden deaths, such as coroner's courts, as well as those religious and funeral professionals dealing with the events following the death, may be the main encounters which the bereaved have with professionals. Thus, workers across the broad spectrum of health and social care, as well as other human services practitioners, are potentially involved to some degree in the care and support of people who are dying and bereaved.

History of care of the dying

Both religious and secular caring professions trace their roots in care of the sick, the wounded and the dying, often citing medieval charitable institutions as the forerunners of modern healthcare, including the hospice movement. In fact, there are some inaccuracies in tracing such links, not least in terms of their sharply divergent philosophical and ideological underpinnings and different focus of care. Medieval European hospices were resting places for those requiring both care and sustenance, taking in as many on account of age, chronic illness and destitution as those who were dying (Clark and Seymour, 1999). In this respect they were similar to later institutions such as, in Britain, the public workhouses set up under the Poor Law Amendment Act of 1834. However, the philosophy of the medieval hospice was rooted in religious and charitable sentiment, unlike the public workhouse, which was concerned with managing those who were a burden on the public purse, and was a fate universally feared. In 1929, a significant piece of legislation, the Local Government Act, separated the Public Health Hospitals from the Public Assistance Institutions, the former providing acute treatments and care for curable conditions, the latter providing care of the old and infirm, and long-term sick. Seen as confirming the establishment of the modern hospital, with priority in terms of both resources and prestige given to the hospitals, some commentators also regard this Act as the beginning of the split between health and social care which we now struggle to integrate (Means and Smith, 1998).

The significance of this history in the care of people who are dying lies in the establishment of competing agendas in public policy:

- The National Health Service was geared towards cure rather than care.
- Long-term public care for incurable conditions was characterised as a burden and linked to economic cost.
- Care based on the values of dignity, love and service was largely preserved through the auspices of religious and voluntary charitable foundations.

This is not to say, as Clark and Seymour (1999) point out, that some of the finest London hospitals, noted for their care of the dying, did not flourish. However, these became focused on the treatment of cancer with priority given to research into more effective curative treatments. It was in this context that the late Cicely Saunders, widely credited with the birth of the modern hospice movement (although St Christopher's in London which she established in 1967 was not the first modern hospice), began her work into the care of dying patients. This has been widely written about elsewhere, including by Dame Saunders herself. For our purposes it is sufficient to note that what was established at St Christopher's, and in the multitude of hospices internationally which sprang up on the same model, were the principles and practice of good *palliative* care (see Chapter Five for discussion of the philosophy and practice of hospice and palliative care). The original hospices were particularly concerned with the relief of pain (physical, emotional and spiritual) and the provision of an environment in which the life of the dying person has value and meaning, and which facilitates a peaceful end. Thus the contemporary notion of 'the good death', which we discuss in Chapter Five, emerged alongside the establishment of palliative care. This was in marked contrast to the prevailing ethos in modern hospitals in the western world, where rapid advances in treatments and success in curing many conditions previously thought incurable, tended to make the dying patient equate with failure for medical and nursing staff, and to lead the patient themselves to feel that they had been abandoned when 'nothing more could be done'. Also established was the principle and practice of holistic care, provided through a multidisciplinary team consisting of medical practitioners, nurses, social workers, occupational and physiotherapists and chaplains, supported by volunteers in capacities ranging from bereavement visiting to running the charity shop.

Hospices have in the main developed through locally raised funding as voluntary organisations, initially all attached to a religious foundation. However, they work alongside statutory services and are therefore affected by changes in health and social care policy and practice, both national directives and local interpretations. Specialist palliative care facilities are also increasing within the NHS. It is to this context which we now turn.

Care management

Care management was introduced in the UK as the framework for health and social care provision to adults in 1993, following the passing of the 1990 National Health Service and Community Care Act (NHSCCA). Care/case management is also the dominant system in North America, Australasia and Hong Kong. Care management is a system for organising service delivery which aims to provide tailored packages of care, based on an individual assessment of need which, if so required by the circumstances of the individual service user, is comprehensive and multidisciplinary and/or multi-agency. The NHSCCA is regarded as a watershed in UK public services provision, and with its objective of producing a 'seamless service' it would seem a wholly appropriate vehicle for meeting the needs of the dying person and their family. However, the introduction of care management has been accompanied by serious questioning in the UK from social work practitioners and academics.

Concerns have been raised about its impact on work with older people (Lymbery, 1998), people with serious illness (Lloyd, 2000) and on the ethos of adult services generally (Lewis and Glennerster, 1996; Cowen, 1999; Lloyd, 2002). Some features of this disquiet have particular implications for work with people who are dying or bereaved. Principally, it is argued that holistic practice is in danger of disappearing (Cowen, 1999); that empowerment falls by the wayside in the face of budget-driven managerialism (Tanner, 1998); that easily measurable service outcomes replace less tangible, relationship-driven or alternative user-defined measures of quality (Nocon and Qureshi, 1996); that it ignores the fact that people ascribe value to means and processes as well as to ends (Priestly, 2000); and that front-line practitioners feel there is no room for the exercise of traditional skills, such as counselling (Lewis and Glennerster, 1996). The threat to holistic practice and counselling skills strikes at the heart of work with people who are dying or bereaved, where it is argued that social workers traditionally brought 'personal and helping skills' to multidisciplinary settings, particularly hospitals (Seden, 1999), and the early hospital social workers (known as 'almoners') established a professional identity based on their use of psychosocial casework (Brearley, 1995).

Although it is social work which has been in the forefront of implementing care management and from which the criticisms have mainly stemmed, the White Paper *Caring for People* (DH, 1989a) was paralleled by its health services equivalent *Caring for Patients* (DH, 1989b). Other professions have also raised concerns about health managerialism triumphing over clinical judgement and the downplaying of professional expertise (Collinson, 1995). Moreover, the trends of marketisation in the caring sector, increasing bureacratisation, managerialism, and de-professionalising influences, with which the implementation of care management in the UK has coincided, are observed to be global and creating similar disquiets in other technologically advanced healthcare systems (Foster and Wilding, 2000).

An individually tailored, coordinated care package sits entirely harmoniously with the provision of holistic care for people who are dying. Ironically, the one model which came to be overwhelmingly adopted by local authorities, the purchaser–provider split, which conceived care management as a series of discrete tasks to be performed by different workers in different parts of the system, is wholly antipathetic to the preserving of holistic practice and the worker–user relationship. In my own research conducted with hospital social workers as they were anticipating the implementation of care management and already experiencing the impact of the shift in underpinning philosophy, workers highlighted organisational constraints as the biggest hindrance to their work and cited the new business culture of health and social care as failing to recognise what they were trying to do (Lloyd, 1997).

Community care legislation has also created other problems. There is no provision in the original guidance to take account of the streamlining of assessment and service delivery processes which is necessary if the needs of dying people are to be met, prompting special pleading from the British Association of Social Workers Palliative Care Special Interest Group to remedy this omission (BASW, 1993). More recently, Nosowska found that people with a terminal illness were missing out on essential benefits because health professionals were failing to advise them early enough, if at all, or to refer them to appropriate sources of information (Nosowska, 2004).

The health and social care interface

The philosophy of holistic care implies that people experience need as whole persons, that although one set of problems may take priority at any one time, the impact is nevertheless felt in all areas of the person's life. This is peculiarly apparent in palliative care, where, for example, although to the professional observer it may seem that the priority is to control the dying person's pain, their 'easeful dying' actually takes place after reunion with a family member. It has long been recognised by policy makers and practitioners that health and social needs overlap, although there is less recognition of the more embracing practice of holistic care, despite rhetoric supporting the concept.

From the mid-1970s, a series of government consultative documents, guidance and directives was issued in the UK, aimed at promoting collaborative arrangements between Health Authorities and Social Services Departments. These concentrated on joint planning and joint finance mechanisms and were prompted by increasing problems of disputed responsibility for care and poor coordination across agencies, which had arisen ever since the 1970 Local Authority Social Services Act and the 1973 National Health Service Reorganisation Act had formally demarcated health care and social care. However, repeated failures in these joint working initiatives lay behind the drive for the reform of community care which took place in the 1990s, a stated government objective being to achieve a 'seamless service' across health and social care.

Thus far, there is everything to applaud in this policy in terms of achieving the best quality care for people who are dying. However, the community care reforms of the 1990s began a focus on achieving cost-effective, streamlined *outcomes*, and away from the machinery of *process*. Service outcomes are measured, not the inputs of different professionals; the emphasis is on their capacity to work together to achieve better health and social welfare outcomes, rather than the different contributions which each makes to the overall care of the service user. There is an obvious tension here with the philosophy of palliative care, built around a model which sees the complementary skills and inputs of different members of the multidisciplinary team as all-important, the best 'outcome' being a death which is as dignified and peaceful as it can be and accords with the wishes of the dying person and their family. In fact, process becomes all-important in achieving this outcome. This does not sit easily within a health and social care system which has favoured easily quantifiable outcomes, such as the numbers of older people supported at home rather than in residential care, and has related these outcomes to easily quantifiable inputs, such as number of patient contacts. Moreover, it actively militates against the ongoing support of the bereaved relative who remains. A community nurse once explained to me that if she spent one hour running a health information group for ten people, she clocked up 10 contacts, whereas if she spent an hour visiting the recently bereaved relative of one of her former patients, it counted as only one. She saw the latter as important, and recognised that it had preventive value in terms of the health and well-being of the bereaved person, but she felt that she was constrained by performance targets which did not value such activity.

The UK modernisation programme

Numerous studies have demonstrated that the care management system has so far failed to deliver the coordinated care which it promised, at sufficient levels of service provision, and to sufficient numbers of people to significantly improve the quality of life and care of most (Lewis et al, 1997; SSI, 1997; Stewart et al, 1999). Thus from 1998 onwards, with first the White Paper *Modernising Social Services* (DH, 1998) and then the 1999 Health Act, the UK government embarked on a strategy of 'modernising services', designed:

- to introduce levers to make progress on collaboration between health and social care agencies, for example additional pooled budgets available only where joint planning processes and service coordination structures can be demonstrated (1999 Health Act);
- to simplify service delivery at the point of contact for the service user, for example the introduction of 'one-stop shops';
- to achieve greater social inclusion and standardisation across user/patient groups and geographical areas, with National Service Frameworks (NSFs) being

developed to regulate standards and procedures for particular groups of service users/patients;

- to modernise the workforce in order to make it 'fit for purpose' in the modernised health and social care system, an emphasis on redefining the 'skills mix' replacing the old professional boundaries (DH, 2002a and b).

As well as a continuing focus on supporting informal carers, particular attention has been given to an integrated assessment process. Among the reasons for the failure of care management to make progress in the integration of health and social care were the obstacles encountered by the local authority charged with the responsibility for procuring a multidisciplinary assessment of need. This was particularly problematic where specialist healthcare assessments were required (Challis et al, 1998). The Single Assessment Process (SAP) is one important measure accompanying the NSF for Older People (DH, 2001), designed to refine referral and assessment systems so as to produce a holistic assessment of need and a comprehensive multidisciplinary response, as and when appropriate, for people over the age of 65. The SAP does not replace community care assessment but is intended to address the latter's failure to achieve an integrated assessment process and to operate within the established care management system.

At the time of writing the success of the modernisation programme has not been fully evaluated. However, three thrusts have emerged which dictate the overall shape of health and social care in the UK:

1. It is to be a *flexible, responsive, 'primary care-led' service*. The move away from institutional care towards care in the community, supporting people to remain living in their own homes or in 'homely settings', for as long as they wish and are able, is now combined with the lead being given to primary care services to ascertain and develop the services to meet the needs of the local community. The local Primary Care Trust (PCT) has the responsibility to commission, purchase and, for some services, directly manage the range of health and social care provision. Whereas under the NHSCCA the lead responsibility lay with the local authority social services department, the lead has effectively transferred back to health for services to adults, although the PCT must contain representatives from, and consult with, all sectors of service provision, including the voluntary sector.
2. It is to offer *person-centred care*, with the expertise of the service user/patient given central importance, and the promotion of independence, autonomy, choice and dignity being overarching objectives. Each of the National Service Frameworks has at its heart this focus on individualised care, underpinned by the above values, encapsulated, for example, in the eight care standards of the NSF for Older People (DH, 2001). The Green Paper *Independence, Well-Being and Choice* (DH, 2004) and its subsequent White Paper *Our Health, Our Care, Our Say* (DH, 2006) bring this together in clear statements about the intended direction and ethos of future health and social care services. Accompanying this is

an emphasis on seeing the service user as the expert on their own situation. This is made most explicit in *The Expert Patient* initiative for the better management of chronic illness (DH, 2000).

3. It is to be a *holistic approach*, understood at the levels of whole systems and whole communities, as well as a whole person approach to the individual 'case' and 'journey'.

The underlying premise of the 'new' approach to interagency collaboration is that health and social care must be holistic, traditionally understood as an approach to individual care which treats 'whole persons'. Under the modernisation of health and social care, 'whole system' changes are seen as the way forward to effect 'whole person' health improvements (Hudson, 2000). This thinking is carried into some of the new roles outlined for the workforce. Particular emphasis is given to an enhanced role for nurses in the community, who are designated as case managers, well-placed to chart and support the patient's overall journey around the health and social care network in the community and across primary and secondary healthcare services (DH, 2005). This is not unlike the role originally envisaged for care managers under the community care system. The difference is that the starting point is health needs rather than everyday living and domiciliary support, although, in theory, both care managers and nurse case managers should be working to a model of comprehensive, holistic assessment, utilising the same range of support services. There is also an emphasis on the management of chronic illness and long-term care or support needs.

Initiatives in palliative care

These global themes in health and social care have particular implications for the development of palliative care. First, the move away from institutional care combined with the objective of maintaining people in their own homes for as long as possible suggests that specialist care for people who are dying should be available in community and homely settings. Second, greater emphasis on supporting people with chronic conditions and the diseases of old age suggests extending the remit of palliative care beyond cancer to other groups who are in the final phase of life but do not have, as such, a 'terminal' diagnosis. This development, combined with increasing numbers of people surviving cancer for five years or more, has contributed to the gradual fading out of the use of the descriptor 'terminal illness'. Third, the emphasis on user expertise and choice, combined with the establishment of the value of empowerment among the caring professions, has challenged palliative care to consider how people who are dying, and their family carers, can be fully involved in their own care and facilitated to exercise choice right to the end. Fourth, the 'person-centred' focus, combined with recognition that some groups have been traditionally excluded or that mainstream services have failed to meet their needs adequately or appropriately, has encouraged hospices and palliative care providers to concentrate on the needs of groups who have been low users of these services. Fifth, the response of the hospice and palliative care movement to the insistence on tangible outcomes, has been greater concentration on, and refinement of, detailed aspects of holistic care, even as the broad principle of holism which it pioneered has received endorsement in mainstream care. Finally, the drive to make boundaries more permeable is putting pressure on hospice care to be a fully integrated part of the health and social care network.

In practice, the process is far less consciously reactive and more reciprocal than this analysis suggests, and, moreover, hospices can be credited with disseminating throughout mainstream services the values of choice, dignity and empowerment in the care of dying people. The strong presence of the voluntary sector in hospice provision has also facilitated the nurturing of bereavement support and family counselling which in statutory services in the UK is generally agreed to be under threat, if not almost extinct. The low-key 'counselling' and emotional support traditionally offered by social workers has been found to be one of the elements that dying and bereaved people value most in all their contacts with professionals (Beresford et al, 2007; Lloyd, 1997). In the US, however, concerns are expressed for the maintenance of psychosocial and spiritual care in end-of-life care programmes, where the funding system dictates that only life-prolonging treatments are reimbursed (Dobratz, 2005). Moreover, it is possible to see recent developments and new directions in palliative care as belonging to the general culture and climate change in health and social care more broadly. These have converged internationally, through the auspices of organisations such as the International Association of Hospice and Palliative Care and the European Association of Palliative Care, in two main directions.

Extension of palliative and hospice care

Whereas at one time hospice care meant care of the patient dying of cancer, current thinking is that the specialist care previously available only in hospices, should be available to every person who has an incurable or life-threatening illness, as soon as they might benefit from it, and in whatever arrangement of service provision best suits their preferences and needs (Rutledge, 2003). In part this has stemmed from the recognition that there are other groups of patients who would benefit from hospice care but with whom the original religious foundation hospices did not feel comfortable – the establishment of specialist hospices for AIDS patients being the most notable example. It has also arisen from a slow recognition that people with other conditions or with significant co-morbidities are frequently denied the benefits of palliative care because they continue to be treated for those diseases rather than simultaneously treated as people who are dying. In the specific case of HIV/AIDS treatment, Harding et al (2005) argue that good palliative care must be *reintroduced* alongside highly active anti-retroviral therapy (HAART) rather than being associated with terminal care. Without this broadened perspective on palliative care, there is evidence of inadequate pain and symptom control for patients with advanced illness, including HIV patients and older people who have suffered a stroke. In 1998, a report commissioned by the National Council for Hospice and Specialist Care Services in the UK highlighted the complex needs of people dying of non-malignant disease and the need for specialist palliative care for people dying of one of the classic conditions of old age. Chapter Six examines the continuing disadvantage experienced by many older people, including their relative exclusion from specialist palliative care facilities. Nevertheless, there is now in the UK and the US widespread acceptance of the need to develop appropriate palliative care for all people with advanced illness. Connolly suggests that this awareness is only just beginning in other parts of Europe and has yet to lead to a policy shift (Connolly, 2003).

One major development has been hospice-at-home schemes, with national associations to promote their development having been set up in a number of countries, including the UK, the US and Australia. Under such schemes, the same technologies and professional care can be provided in the home as are available in the specialist palliative care unit in the hospital or the hospice. As well as 'hands-on care', professionals will offer information and advice for both patients and informal carers. This potentially covers the full spectrum of professional inputs, from pain and symptom control and medication management, to dietary advice, occupational and physiotherapy to improve comfort and ease of daily living, to emotional support and psychological counselling. However, for some people, home ceases to feel like home if it is overrun by professionals or becomes too like the high-tech hospital, and therefore they prefer institutional care, at least for the last days or weeks (Gott et al, 2004).

In general, the trend to move palliative care out into the community relies on a flexible use of support and treatment services, including periods spent as a hospital in-patient, day attendance at hospices or hospital units, and primary care and community health and social care services working in conjunction with specialist palliative care services. There is also an increasing trend for hospice admission to occur later in the illness, sometimes only for a few days, so that it is effectively part of the community care network. The palliative care needs of people in nursing home care are also recognised, including the particular needs of those with degenerative conditions such as Parkinson's disease (Thomas, 2006) and Alzheimer's (Haak, 2004). A pilot project in South Wales adapted the concept of intermediate care[1] to set up a palliative care unit within a nursing home. The evaluation suggested that such units have the potential to increase the options available to service users and remove the necessity for residents of registered care homes to face the disruption of hospital admission in the last few weeks of life (Saysell, 2004).

In these community initiatives, the role of the family doctor is crucial. A study in the UK found that 73 per cent of the patients who died in a rural GP practice between July 1998 and June 2000, died whilst under the direct care of their family doctor (Mitchell and Seamark, 2003). This has implications for the training of general practitioners, with patients in some studies expressing anxieties that pain control would not be as good at home as in a hospital or hospice (Gott et al, 2004). In the UK, an initiative to establish a lead clinician for cancer in each PCT has been welcomed as significantly improving and standardising palliative care offered by the primary care team (Leese et al, 2004). Evaluations of the role of home care services and community nurses have suggested that primary care practitioners welcome the opportunity to provide palliative care for patients at home (for example, Hanley, 2004; Wilkes and White, 2005), but the quality of the service which can be offered is dependent on straightforward and equal access to specialist services (Todd et al, 2002). A US study found that hospices did not always fit easily into the care continuum, particularly for patients receiving complex palliative treatments, who might be excluded from some hospices because of inadequate clinical capacity (Lorenz et al, 2004). At the same time, it is argued that hospice and palliative care services are leading the way in the concept and practice of integrated care services (Howell, 2004).

Crucially, the success of the extension of palliative care into the community, and across the spectrum of healthcare provision, depends on the effective integration of health and social care and multiprofessional initiatives. In the US, progress is reported to be slow, with people with life-limiting illness still forced to choose between curative treatments or comfort care (Reb, 2003). A UK/US cross-national secondary review of the evidence concerning access to HIV/AIDS palliative care (Harding et al, 2005) recommended that the barriers found would only be addressed by:

- multiprofessional assessment, able to engage with the heterogeneous needs of the minority populations that are overwhelmingly affected by HIV, and which leads to a response informed by understanding of social inequality and discrimination;
- palliative care training given to all practitioners and clinicians, and palliative care domains included in all standard assessments;
- the development and refinement of referral systems to cope with complex palliative care needs, including better communication between palliative care and HIV specialists;
- better training of palliative care staff so that they understand the breadth of palliative care need as it relates to advanced HIV disease.

Similar conclusions are drawn by Seymour et al (2005) in their report on end-of-life care for older people, particularly where they have a complex illness such as advanced Parkinson's disease. The UK government is rolling out an end-of-life care programme aimed at establishing four tools to address this agenda:

- 'Building on the Best, Choice, Responsiveness and Equity' – a training strategy aimed at ensuring all adults at the end of life have access to staff trained in end-of-life care;

- The Gold Standards Framework – aimed particularly at helping GPs to plan with patients, their families and other professionals in their last six to nine months of life for the care which they are likely to need and wish to have;
- The Liverpool Care Pathway – to be used in the last days or hours of life and aimed at transferring the best of hospice care into hospitals and other care settings;
- The Preferred Place of Care – an advanced care plan retained by patients as they move through different care settings, indicating and updating their choices including where they want to be when they die.

Palliative care in multicultural contexts

Alongside the criticism which accompanied the AIDS epidemic in the 1980s of hospices as being too overtly religious, questions were raised about the lack of take-up of hospice places by people from ethnic minority groups. Recent reports commissioned by the National Council for Hospices and Specialist Palliative Care Services (NCHSPCS, 1995 and 2001) indicate that progress continues to be slow on this issue in the UK. Nyatanga suggests that the position is worse in the UK than other western countries (Nyatanga, 2002); nevertheless, recent evidence from the US shows African-Americans, Hispanics and Asians trailing behind white beneficiaries of Medicare in their use of hospice services (Miller and Ryndes, 2005). The NCHSPCS reports found a continuing surprisingly low take-up of cancer and specialist palliative care services by people from black and minority ethnic groups. Some of the reasons for this appear to relate to a lack of knowledge about these services (Ahmed et al, 2004; Payne et al, 2006) but also to the fact that they are less likely to be referred, and once referred, tend to make less use of such services (Ahmed et al, 2004). Thus a further angle of interest for researchers has been to explore what sort of care is wanted by different ethnic groups, and what is meant by culturally competent practice.

The point is made many times in this book that the subject of death and dying lends itself too easily to a 'list' approach to different cultures and religions, cataloguing people's needs according to the main beliefs and practices of the culture to which they ostensibly belong, whereas the needs of the individual, particularly those living in multicultural or cross-cultural situations, demand a much greater depth of understanding and tailored response. There has been a repeated tendency to refer to 'black and ethnic minority groups' as though they are one homogeneous category of people. In fact, not only is there significant religious and cultural heterogeneity even within groups such as the Chinese in the UK (Payne et al, 2005), there are also significant differences in their economic and social circumstances, both within and across groups (DH, 1999).

Progress in delivering culturally appropriate services and culturally competent practice cannot therefore take place without a critical understanding of 'culture'. Moreover, the issues are especially sensitive in palliative care since the management of death is embedded in social structures and the individual response is determined by an inextricable intertwining of psychological, social and philosophical factors. We cannot begin to practise competently if we do not engage with differences in beliefs about health, illness, dying and death (Gatrad and Sheikh, 2002; Nyatanga, 2002).

There is a valuable critique building of the meanings of 'culture' and its application to the development of services and professional practice. First, it is pointed out that the term 'ethnic minority community' can signify a valuing of difference, but it can also be used to confirm 'otherness' (Owens and Randhawa, 2004), particularly where staff show little understanding of issues of cultural identity and, for example, the reasons for dietary requests (Gunaratnam, 2001). Second, the principles of hospice and palliative care may be advertised globally but may be variously interpreted in different countries, and the concepts underpinning the principles may have different meanings (Nyatanga, 2002). It should not be assumed that palliative care as conceived in western countries would universally be regarded as a 'good thing' – indeed, some of its objectives may not transfer easily across cultures (Owens and Randhawa, 2004). The notion of the individual patient at the centre of their own care, and the person with whom the professional communicates first and foremost, might be one such instance where practice could actually prove counter-cultural, particularly where there are also gender and age cultural imperatives to take into account. Third, anti-discriminatory assessment requires a sensitive engagement with the subjective experience of the individual within their cultural context, as much for the person belonging to an ethnic minority as for anyone else (Gunaratnam et al, 1998). Gunaratnam accuses service providers of both 'cultural reductionism' and 'cultural and religious prescription' in their attempts to address the needs of ethnic minority patients in palliative care (Gunaratnam, 1997). Fourth, religion and spirituality are confirmed as extremely important dimensions of palliative care practice in multicultural contexts. However, the concept of transcultural spirituality, involving the search to establish and access shared meaning, may provide a more helpful framework for the development of empathic practice than 'multicultural' approaches which can emphasise 'otherness' in their eagerness to recognise difference (Holloway, 2006a).

Finally, and this applies to the whole of health and social care services, the notion of ethnic minorities 'looking after their own', informal caring being the automatic choice of families who are themselves supported within an extended family and community, has been repeatedly challenged but is an attitude still displayed by practitioners. UK studies have shown that the reality for many carers from minority communities is that the model of the lone, socially isolated carer predominates, their problems frequently compounded by racial harassment, the carer's ill-health and poverty (McCalman, 1990). Ethnic minority carers' contacts with formal services continue to be frequently at very low levels (Owens and Randhawa, 2004), perhaps indicating the prevalence of the view from service providers that their support is not needed. Moreover, traditions of 'filial piety' are increasingly being overturned through the concern of aged parents not to be a burden on economically active and socially mobile children (Chapman et al, 2005).

Conclusion

Despite significant differences in the organisation and funding of health and social care systems in the west, their broad directions and the issues raised are remarkably similar. Most notably, there is a move away from attention to process and a focus on the outcomes of care. This sits uneasily with the philosophy of hospice and palliative care. In the US, where many health insurance schemes do not fund palliative care, there is concern that end-of-life care is being forced into blurring 'curing' and 'caring' treatments and the essential spirit of palliative care may be lost (Dobratz, 2005). In the UK, a House of Commons Select Committee inquiry into palliative care services has resulted in a cash boost for hospice organisations, with ring-fenced monies for both end-of-life care for older people and children's hospices. While this is to be welcomed, the funds are hedged by requirements for them to be spent on capital investment programmes and 'tangible physical environmental improvements'. Internationally, there is a shortage of consultants in palliative medicine and specialist nurses in palliative care. The effects of this are being felt in continuing poor symptom control and in palliative care being offered far too late, if at all (Allen, 2004; Miller and Ryndes, 2005). The history of palliative care has demonstrated that 'best value' is achieved through skilled multidisciplinary intervention with the practitioner's time and emotional support being as important as any aspect of the physical environment. Only thus, with time spent ensuring the dignity and comfort of the dying person, and enabling them, and their families, to exercise choice and control in their situation, can the only outcome which really matters – a death which is as they wish it – take place. It is likely that palliative care is going to have to fight to maintain its particular interpretation of these objectives on the policy agenda.

What of the care and support of people bereaved through whatever circumstance? The future of dedicated counselling services looks patchy overall and precarious in any state-funded or insurance-funded system. The flourishing of bereavement theory in the US and northern Europe would suggest that grief counselling is going on at sufficient levels to stimulate this theoretical development, but it is an educated guess that this is largely in private practice. In the UK, those individuals and families who struggle particularly with complicated grief and who are able to make their pain heard by their doctor, may be referred to clinical psychologists or counsellors attached to GP practices. Voluntary organisations exist for the support of bereaved parents, widows, suicide survivors and a range of specific diseases. Bereavement support is offered by most religious professionals performing funeral services, but will not, for the most part, be ongoing. The lay community may in general be more sensitised to the needs of recently bereaved people, but this support tends to fade quickly away and for those people who are socially marginalised or isolated, their contacts with routine health and social care services, however fleeting, may be the only opportunity for their grief to be acknowledged and responded to. Bereavement support is unlikely to become a policy priority in the health and social care systems of the twenty-first century.

Death, however, increasingly figures in those encounters. Thus the *way* in which the person-to-person encounter is managed is, as the hospice mission originally realised, of crucial importance if health and social care services are to address the needs of dying and bereaved persons across the board. Chapter Eight looks in further detail at that challenge for the different professions which make up the mosaic of contemporary care.

Note

[1] Intermediate care is one initiative within the UK government's modernising services programme which aims to provide the additional treatment and support of hospital or residential care facilities within the community for people who require them as a short-term measure, thus preventing hospital or residential admissions.

THREE

Understanding death and dying

Introduction

Death, dying and bereavement have been the subject of considerable interest to scholars since the middle of the twentieth century, despite the message that we are a 'death-denying' society. These attempts to understand how death is handled in societies and its impact on individuals and communities become ever more complex as one dominant approach supersedes another, or new refinements in relation to particular categories of bereavement are suggested. Despite differences in emphasis and divides in opinion, at the heart of these developments lies the widely accepted assumption that dying and bereavement are experiences which are both individually and socially mediated. Thus, as societies change, it is likely that dying and bereavement will be experienced differently by individuals, yet the psychological phenomena of attachment and loss may remain essentially unchanged. In fact, we still know remarkably little about the interaction between the individual subjective experience of loss and the particular social system to which that individual belongs.

A number of disciplines have contributed to this theorising and each makes its own contribution at the same time as it has something to say about the whole picture. So, for example, in the early part of the twentieth century, it was social anthropology which turned its attention to the rituals and symbols which societies construct to manage death, first through the examination of primitive societies but then shifting focus to search for the patterns in modern society. The degree to which social ritual is present or absent around death has been taken up by sociologists as a key indicator of whether or not death is denied, hidden or open in a given society. The denial of death became a central tenet in sociologists' accounts of death in modern western societies. If death is avoided in the public gaze, how does the individual cope with the painful experience of loss occasioned by a significant bereavement? Psychologists and psychiatrists began to use not just biological explanations to explain grief but also to look for social determinants which might exacerbate or alleviate distress. And more recently, grief counsellors have rediscovered the therapeutic power of ritual and symbolism.

Two ancient disciplines have remained largely outside this cross-fertilisation of ideas. Theology and philosophy have been interested in death and its relationship to life from the outset. Yet the contributions of both have been almost wholly neglected by British sociologists in the twentieth-century study of death. This may be due to the predominant view that the UK is a profoundly secular society and religion is of little continuing relevance, let alone theological discourse. The

American thanatology movement has been rather more inclined to include both religion and theology within its orbit. Moreover, the growing interest in spirituality and spiritual care, combined with a recognition that 'faith' (be that religious or humanistic) plays an important part in the management of their dying and bereavement for significant numbers of individuals and growing sectors of our ethnically diverse societies, also points to a need to revise the secularisation of death thesis. Secularisation, however, does not account for the neglect (aside from selected contributions on medical ethics) of philosophy. It is part of the argument of this book that, as the Oxford philosopher, Mary Midgely, expressed in a BBC radio interview some years ago, if philosophy is viewed as the plumbing of society, then the 'bad smell' of late modernity has arisen from society's failure to maintain its plumbing system! The current issues facing advanced health and social care systems in their management of life and death have in common philosophical and ethical dimensions with which we are simply not used to wrestling – or, at any rate, our capacity to do something has run ahead of our thinking about whether we *should* or might wish to do so. To a limited extent, this chapter and the next will seek to integrate perspectives on death from theology and philosophy, as well as approaches to understanding dying and bereavement from pastoral theology.

Death as a phenomenon is of interest to sociologists and anthropologists in terms of how it is managed in society, to psychologists in terms of the attitudes which individuals hold towards death, to philosophers in terms of the demarcation of human existence, and to theologians in terms of the implications for life. One of the consequences of this analysis has been the attempts to model and typify death. Before looking in detail at some of these, let us briefly touch on the work of the French social historian, Philippe Aries, since his analysis tracing changing European attitudes to death since the Middle Ages, treating death as a social event which represents itself through symbolic ritual, has provided something of a prototype (Aries, 1974). It is Aries' description of death in the twentieth century which has been most influential. Death in modern western (Protestant) societies is described as 'forbidden death'. Significant criticisms have been made of Aries' scholarship, but his description of the twentieth century as a death-denying society has been influential in the development of the modern death thesis.

Beliefs, ritual and symbolism

It is in the study of rituals and symbols that we find the greatest attempts to theorise the practices associated with death. There are two essays which are generally regarded as seminal works in the anthropological literature and still referred to in recent writings, such as Seale's sociological account of dying and bereavement (Seale, 1998). The combined work of Hertz and Van Gennep established a theoretical framework, which has been repeatedly applied to the study of death rites and rituals in societies and cultures as diverse as a Pacific Island and America in the 1960s.

Rites of passage

Although published slightly later than Hertz's 1907 essay on 'secondary burial', Van Gennep's essay in 1909 (translated into English in 1960), entitled *The Rites of Passage*, laid the foundation for considering ritual as a device for managing life's major transitions, which shares a common structure, purpose and function. It has been hugely influential. Van Gennep's core concept is that each state has two categories which are directly opposed – for example, alive/dead – and that the passing from one to the other takes place in three stages: separation from the first status, followed by a liminal phase before integration into the new status. Each stage is marked by rites which facilitate the transition and which incorporate opposing symbols. So, for example, death rites are concerned with symbols of decay/degeneration and fertility/regeneration. Metcalfe and Huntington argue that the importance of Van Gennep's contribution is that he made 'ritual everywhere accessible to a similar logic' (Metcalfe and Huntington, 1991, p. 31). In their own edited volume, these symbols are extensively explored in societies past and present, primitive and modern.

Establishing a liminal state

The concept and embodiment of rites of passage contain within them a stage which is finding increasing currency in the analysis of contemporary death – the liminal state. The concept of liminality was introduced by anthropologists to explore how societies dealt with the transition from life to death, using it as an explanation for the period of time after death during which certain rituals were performed after which the deceased could be regarded as 'finally dead'. In a collection of essays exploring the management of death in late medieval and early modern Europe, Gordon and Marshall (2000) explain how these peoples determined the social and ontological status of the dead and why they needed to do so. In circumstances where death rates were dramatically higher than experienced in comparative societies currently, and life expectancy was considerably lower with high rates of infant mortality, the phenomenon of 'social death', in which the dying person is prematurely cut off from the living as if they were already dead, did not exist. The problem was not, as presently, how to prevent the marginalisation and disengagement of older people but how to incorporate the 'social presence' of the recently dead. Thus we see considerable emphasis on those rites and rituals which marked the transition from the status of 'alive' to that of 'dead'. The really interesting point of comparison with contemporary societies is the consistent need to establish a liminal state. Van Gennep himself had emphasised that funeral rituals throughout the world were more associated with liminality than with moving on and letting go. More recent scholarship from sociologists has suggested that in late modernity the stage between life and death is again more evident, this time experienced in the prolongation of life brought about by people living longer, assisted by improved health and healthcare and, in some cases, wholly dependent upon medical technology. The problem now is how society manages a liminal state which occurs before, rather than after, biological death. We explore this further in Chapter Six.

Why should it be any more difficult for contemporary societies to manage this liminal state in life than it was for the peoples of medieval Europe to structure the gradual 'letting go' of their dead? One clue may lie in the relationship between rite, ritual and belief. Returning to the anthropologists, Hertz developed the notion of secondary burial as marking the ending of the liminal state. Hertz described rituals which accommodated a period in which the individual was neither alive nor finally treated as dead. During this period both the community left behind and the dead person have to achieve that final separation, which for the latter involves the soul being released from the corpse. Hertz postulated that the practice of exhumation and secondary disposal of the corpse allowed the living to satisfy themselves that this transition phase, in which the soul was discomforted and potentially a threat to the living, was at an end.

As Metcalfe and Huntington point out, the practice of secondary burial is surprisingly widespread. What is even more common, and historically highly significant as a shaper of death rites and funeral practices, is the underpinning belief system of the duality of body and soul, in which the soul at death enters a transitory phase before its final fate, or resting place, is determined. This may involve the continuing existence of the disembodied soul, or the generation of a new life or existence out of the death and decay of the previous one. Christian theologians trace the origins of this thinking to Plato and church historians have extensively documented the associated practices, such as praying for the dead and purchasing indulgences, around beliefs in Purgatory and resurrection. Belief in ghosts, although in direct contradiction to Christian belief, has coexisted with it throughout Europe from medieval times to the present day, where it sustains a surprising degree of popular interest (Caciola, 2000). Such beliefs may become personalised for the individual bereaved relative, as the following quotation from my own research illustrates:

> 'It's like he's wandering about up there. I don't think he has settled ... it scares me.' (Lloyd, 1996, p 306)

Social historians have examined periods in which society and religion are inextricably entwined. They demonstrate that rites and rituals go hand in hand with the beliefs which support them and without which the symbols fall into disuse. Thus, in periods of seismic change, such as the English Reformation, the rites of passage were fundamentally affected (for example, prayers for the dead faded away) creating considerable instability among the common people until beliefs and practices eventually reharmonised (Coster, 2000). Thus far, there is little research into contemporary beliefs about death held by people in developed countries despite the common assertion that contemporary culture is more or less secular. The suggestion that an extended old age and artificially sustained life is creating a liminal phase *before* death presents us with a problem when we note that the liminal state is universally constructed through rite and ritual. In contemporary society, we have not yet established the appropriate rituals to assist either the living or the dying to negotiate this 'dying phase' of life.

Immortality and regeneration

Another important belief underpinning secondary burial practices is the notion of new life arising from the ashes of the old. This accounts for the prevalence of fertility rites in the burial practices of many primitive cultures. Often, these rituals include a sacrificial element. Again, this is a rite inextricably linked to its underpinning beliefs. Christianity, for example, contains at its heart the death of Christ as the supreme sacrifice that gives new life to humankind. Each of the world's major religions contains within it belief in resurrection, reincarnation or immortality of the soul, in each case achieved through the 'throwing off' of the 'mortal coil'. Popular folklore also contains similar themes; there is still some evidence of people believing that an older member will die when a new baby joins the family ('one in, one out'). However, many people in advanced, secularised societies nowadays are neither religious nor superstitious, or, if still broadly in sympathy with a particular religious belief system, have only a hazy adherence to its traditional position on death and a life thereafter. Yet the themes we have touched on here are sufficiently widespread and long-standing in burial and funeral rites to suggest that they might endure beyond the radical transformation of the belief culture. It may be that what is being asserted is the continuance of life in the face of death. Some have gone further and suggested that in contemporary society we refuse to relinquish control to death (Grainger, 1998).

This is an idea which finds currency in recent studies. Young and Cullen, from their study of terminally ill cancer patients in East London, pursue the idea of 'a collective immortality' (Young and Cullen, 1996). They argue that people demonstrated a need for a sense of continuity between the dead and the living and were searching for mechanisms which reinforce that. They suggest that funeral and burial practices would benefit from revision to create rituals which acknowledge the continuing contribution of those who have gone before, both individuals and passing generations or eras, to the continuance of life as it is now. The need for this continuity was variously expressed by the people in my own research, but most strongly by those who did not hold a firm religious faith but were searching to establish or maintain a meaningful connection for themselves. Implicit in these statements is the belief that there is something else that does continue, described by some of the people in my research as 'spiritual bonding' (Lloyd, 1996). At its most basic, the desire for a deceased relative or friend to be missed and remembered by a community is common among grieving persons.

The regenerative power of the encounter with death creating a new outlook on life, new direction, sometimes almost a new person, which is often expressed in our society, clearly echoes the themes of rebirth and new life which feature so strongly in traditional death rituals. Perhaps the question with which we must grapple is whether we need new rituals to express and confirm these themes, and, if so, what they should be. There is evidence of the translation of these themes into contemporary funeral, disposal and memorial practices (see Chapter Seven) but as yet these 'alternative' practices are marked by diversity and also some disorganisation as the attempts to personalise and recreate ritual leaves much to the individual at a time of great stress. Such questions are thrown into sharp relief when alongside the affirmation of life, our technological age also controls the manner and moment of death.

Modern death

The study of death emerged as a new avenue for sociological enquiry in the mid-twentieth century. A growing body of work, each strand having a slightly different focus, coalesced to produce a picture of contemporary death in the western world which became the accepted wisdom in both academic analysis and the caring professions. In contrast to pre-modern societies where death was common and accepted as part of life, these analysts argued that in the modern world, death is no longer experienced 'in the midst of life', and that the social rituals attending death and the expected period of mourning have been reduced to almost nothing. This widespread 'denial of death' lies behind the huge difficulties experienced by individuals in their grief (Gorer, 1965). A second theme is that the removal of death from everyday life is compounded by the environment of the modern hospital where most people die, their dying controlled by professionals who manage death behind a technical barrage and impersonal bureaucracy. Death itself is shrouded in silence, and dying and bereaved persons are left isolated and unsupported (for example, Hinton, 1967, 1980; Aries, 1974, 1981; Elias, 1985). Traditional ways of managing death are replaced, meanwhile, by a professionalised funeral industry, which seeks to make death more palatable and sanitised for modern consumption (Mitford, 1963 and 2000). The 'modern death' thesis has for some time now been subject to revision, but there are separate elements within it which are worth considering in more depth, not least because they appear to be surviving into late modernity, albeit adapted to the changed context.

Death as taboo

First, the notion of death as a taboo subject, with its attendant combination of silent disapproval and prurient expression, was first highlighted by the British sociologist, Geoffrey Gorer. Gorer termed death the new 'pornography' and introduced the idea of the *stigma* of grief (Gorer, 1965). The stigma of terminal illness, as well as the stigma experienced by bereaved people, continues to be identified (for example, Snidle, 1996; Lloyd, 1997; Chan et al, 2000)

> 'They're very embarrassed, when you're talking about it, because if I see a person I haven't seen for a good while, they say, "how're you

> doing?" I say, "Well, apart from the cancer I'm alright." Oh, they step back a bit.' (Female, author's previously unreported data)

However, there is a subtle twist to Gorer which can almost be seen as a direct corollary of improved treatments for cancer and even of developments in palliative care. If we cannot cure with treatment, we heal through care, and death itself remains the taboo. Respondents in my own research (Lloyd, 1996 and 1997) who were hospice patients pointed out that although there was much talk about cancer in the hospice, no one mentioned death: 'We can talk about cancer, quite open. But death, no. That's the only down thing about this place' (female patient, author's own previously unreported data).

Campione, a leading Italian doctor in hospice care, describes Italian hospices as places where death is not talked about, but must be fought against; the quest for healing replaces the engagement with death. Campione argues that this is the only philosophy which allows hospices to be integrated into Italian culture and society (Campione, 2004).

Other work has taken the pornography argument further, asserting that late modernity is fascinated by death but must sensationalise it. The frequent coverage in the popular media is sometimes taken as evidence that as a society we have overcome our reluctance to talk about death. However, Pickering et al (1997) argue that postmodernity is unable to deal with death without contradictions and crassness. Walter (one of the members of this research team) in an earlier discussion of death as taboo suggests that at the very least a lot of people continue to approach it as such in popular culture. He offers a number of modifications to the taboo theory, including that it is mainly among health professionals that death is the unmentionable (Walter, 1991). Quoting their own study which looked at coverage of death in the media, Pickering et al (1997) describe the media's representation as 'death's public sting', reporting that during a three-month period in 1992, death stories featured on 41.5 per cent of all newspaper front pages. However, this was the shocking yet salacious face of public death – murders, child suicide, celebrity deaths. This seems to echo the early contention of Glaser and Strauss (1965) that attitudes to death were paradoxical, most Americans preferring to talk about particular deaths of strangers whilst continuing to avoid the phenomenon of death itself or the deaths of people close to themselves.

Death as several deaths

A second sub-theme is the idea of death as a fragmented phenomenon. No longer is death a single event but made up of a number of smaller deaths. Aries describes it thus:

> Death is a technical phenomenon obtained by a cessation of care ... Death has been dissected, cut to bits by a series of little steps, which finally makes it impossible to know which step was the real death ...

> All these little silent steps have replaced and erased the dramatic act of death. (Aries, 1981, p 88)

Thus we can distinguish 'biological death', that is, physical cessation, from 'social death', where the individual gradually ceases to exist as a social being (Sudnow, 1967), and a further distinction, which I shall term 'personal death', involves the loss of personhood. The manifestations of these 'little deaths' are becoming more complex and also more intertwined. Much of this stems from advances in medical technology, which raise ethical questions for both society in general and professional caregivers in particular, which are the subject of Chapter Five. Personhood is frequently equated with the capacity to reason and act autonomously and arguments about loss of personhood and independent functioning are used to determine at which point in the physical deterioration life has effectively ceased. Social death may occur as the dying individual becomes cut off from communication and interaction with other people, in part because of their own body shutting down and in part because of the way in which they are treated by those around them. Ainsworth-Smith and Speck (1982) describe this process as narrowing 'cones of awareness', in which the dying person's interactions become increasingly limited. To counter this, the hospice movement has emphasised that people *live* until they die (Saunders, 1990). Social death may also occur as a particular individual or group becomes unwillingly isolated, marginalised and cut off from the mainstream. This social exclusion all too frequently results in health inequalities and 'disadvantaged dying'. Chapter Six focuses on the experiences of death for older people, for whom the cumulative effect of biological, social and personal death may be an intensely stigmatising and isolating experience.

Another feature of the modern death picture highlighted by Aries is termed 'privatised death'. The point is not that people necessarily die alone, but that death procedures are taken over by impersonal bureaucracies or professionals and the subjective experience for both the dying person and bereaved relatives has to be faced without the nurture of community. Elias (1985) makes clear that it is the necessity for dying and bereaved individuals to make sense of their experiences alone which creates the loneliness. The extent to which death remains privatised in today's society is one of the aspects of the modern death thesis which has been called into question and this book is particularly concerned with the ways in which 'public' and 'private' are being redefined. However, a number of the features of privatised death remain:

- 'Private grief' is regarded as a dignified, civilised process, and it is a cultural myth that all non-western cultures encourage loud wailing.
- Many people are alone at the point of death, either in institutional care or at home, where the body may remain undiscovered for some time if the person lived alone.
- Many funerals and burials are confined to the immediate family, although there may be a memorial service later.

- The dead body is taken over by the mortuary or funeral parlour and often viewed only by closest relatives, if at all.

Not only is death privatised, it is argued that it is *prettified* and made more acceptable to modern society. In a scathing description of the American funeral industry, Jessica Mitford exposed the prettifying of death as an appendage of life, with elaborate embalming techniques including suntans and makeovers, funeral parlours becoming 'plush palaces of death'. As traditional rituals faded, the old symbols of death were replaced by new symbolic practices belonging to modern consumerist society, like 'pre-need selling' of funeral packages and 'not-yet-dead' lists. An equally disturbing update on this prettifying of death is provided in Lawton's account of 'dirty dying'. Arguing from a participant observation study, Lawton suggests that hospice care has moved imperceptibly away from opening up dying to being a vehicle for the sequestration of death, in particular, the shunting out of sight of the wholly unpalatable deaths in which deterioration of the body is out of control (Lawton, 1998). Chapter Seven provides further evidence of the ways in which contemporary funeral and disposal practices are finding ever more varied ways of making death more acceptable to the living.

Secularisation

A core theme in the modern death analysis is the argument that western societies have become progressively secularised. The decline in organised religion is cited as a major factor in the reduction of traditional practices and ritual and, hence, the removal of a traditional source of support for individuals and, for those individuals who do not subscribe to an established belief system, a means of understanding death. Mitford (1963) declared that capitalism had replaced religion in death and professional funeral directors had become the new clergy, shepherding the bereaved through replacement rituals. As with other elements of the modern death analysis, this crude picture has been subject to revision and more complex elaboration. There is no doubt that church attendances in northern Europe have declined in the second half of the twentieth century (they remain significantly higher in the US) although exact figures are difficult to obtain and even more difficult to analyse conclusively when regional factors, differences between economic centres and rural areas, age, gender and class variations, not to mention the complexities of immigrant and ethnic minority populations, are taken into account (Bruce, 1995). Bruce attributes this secularisation primarily to the social consequences of modernisation, individualism and the decline in community having deprived the church of its social role. He dismisses arguments that human beings display enduring religious need, by arguing that such needs will only be framed in a religious manner in a religious society. It is only in those 'dark recessive areas' where technology has not yet triumphed that people in the modern world turn to religion.

Thus, the findings of studies into death and dying, which continue to feature religious faith and practice as an important dynamic, and ministers of religion as having a significant social role, would presumably be viewed as describing a phenomenon that will diminish over time. Seale and Cartwright found only one in six bereaved relatives reporting that they and the deceased had *no* religious faith, and over 90 per cent of those with strong religious faith reporting it to have been helpful (Seale and Cartwright, 1994). However, among the old, religious faith was more common. Reflecting on this higher reporting of religious faith than in general attitude surveys, Seale and Cartwright comment that it could be explained by the skewing towards old age in their sample, or 'it could be that both approaching death and experience of bereavement stimulate religious belief' (1994, p 61).

This was certainly the case in my own study, where the majority had not been regular church attenders during their adult lives but demonstrated some sort of 'religious sense' (Lloyd, 1997). Bruce argues that in modern societies we see increasing secularisation and loss of specific religious beliefs but a continuing 'fondness for vague religious affirmations' (Bruce, 1995, p. 51).

The revival of death

In the late twentieth century a revision of the picture of modern death emerges. Tony Walter is credited with first using the phrase 'revival of death' (Walter, 1994), and while not all subsequent work follows Walter's initial line, it does argue that the ways in which individuals and societies deal with death in late modernity are more diverse than earlier analyses had allowed. If there is a denial of death, it is not necessarily in the form of hidden or forbidden death. Walter suggests a typology of *traditional death*, *modern death* and *postmodern death* as 'ideal types' (Walter, 1994). Each 'ideal type' is located in particular cultural and historical contexts and provides an entry for exploring the meanings of death, rather than a model as such. Although Walter argues that aspects of each type coexist, there is a general historical drift.

Postmodern death

Postmodern theorists argue that the long-accepted description of modern death no longer holds true. Contemporary approaches to death are characterised by plural identities, redrafting of the self, and in a social context in which the boundaries between life and death are more diffuse. Walter is particularly concerned with two aspects: bereavement and funerals. He proclaims that the grief counsellors and professionals have taken over dying and bereavement on a grand scale and are out of step with the thoughts, feelings and modes of expression of ordinary bereaved people. Walter goes on to assert that individuals are concerned to control their own dying and bereavement. However, when it comes to funerals, Walter argues that we have not yet achieved the same degree of personal customisation as in our management of bereavement, mainly because the 'postmodern self' is short on the resources on which to draw to replace the functions and purposes of traditional rituals. Quoting Giddens he argues that we have replaced ritual with discourse – and 'talk' tends to focus on the life lived and the lives remaining, rather than the social and existential transition of death, particularly when belief structures are absent. Chapter Seven further analyses the impact of this on the shape of secular funerals.

Two immediate responses must be made to Walter's thesis. First, as Small (1997) has pointed out, there is something of a contradiction in constructing an ideal postmodern type. Walter's exhortation to individuals to find their own ways of dealing with death nevertheless represents an attempt to contain and routinise death, and we have to ask ourselves why we continue to feel this need. Second, there is plenty of evidence to suggest that individuals are eager to embrace 'given' models and structures to help them understand death – part of the appeal of 'stage theory' to bereaved people and their counsellors (see Chapter Four) was that it seemed to be right in retrospect, as much as whilst in the throes of grief, it seemed to be too neat. Arnason and Hafsteinsson (2003) argue from the experience of CRUSE[1] that the main thrust of bereavement counselling in the community has been to listen to the client as expert on their own experience and assist them in objectifying and codifying that experience. In my research I found that dying and bereaved individuals were anxious to establish and draw on a wider belief framework in which to locate their subjective experience (Lloyd, 1996). The extensive and continuing work on complicated grief discussed in Chapter Four would, arguably, be unsustainable, if coping with grief was simply a matter of individuals having the confidence to follow their own instincts.

Death both absent and present

At the centre of the revision of modern death lies the question of whether, and to what extent, societies in late modernity are death-denying. Kellehear (1984) proposed that the arguments do not hold up from a sociological viewpoint. Seale (1998) agrees with Kellehear, commenting that, far from being death-denying, modern industrialised societies have actively organised themselves to accommodate and deal with death. However, Seale distinguishes between sociological and psychological denial, his central thesis being that social and cultural life, almost by definition, involves a turning away from death and affirmation of life. Sociologists use the term 'sequestration' to refer to the processes and strategies used by societies to avoid direct confrontation with death. However, Smith argues that the very processes of avoiding and concealing death require organisation at individual and communal levels which implies that death is never far from our thinking and omnipresent in our social organisation: 'death is both absent and present' (Smith, 2006, p 225). The poet, Philip Larkin, expresses the same sentiment:

> In time the curtain-edges will grow light.
> Till then I see what's really always there:
> Unresting death …
> …
> It stands plain as a wardrobe, what we know,
> Have always known, know that we can't escape,
> Yet can't accept. One side will have to go.[2]

Smith utilises actor network theory, suggesting that our connections with death are organised through a network of elements – social, technological and physical. He proposes that when this invisible network is disrupted, death as raw confrontation breaks through. So, for example, parents of children treated at the Alder Hey hospital in Liverpool, England, who discovered after the burial that organs had been removed, without their permission, from the dead bodies of their babies, had their recollections, remembrances and memorials so disrupted that in some cases they felt driven to bury their baby again. Whether or not we agree with Smith's theory, what his example illustrates is the importance *and visibility* which continues to be accorded to the physical body and its disposal in our secular, technological society.

The phenomenon of 'privatised death' has also been questioned. Some researchers suggest that the picture of privatised death has never been as widespread as originally thought, or has been only partially true, particularly in rural and more traditional communities (Williams, 1990; Clark, 1993). Alternatively, it is suggested that people nowadays have developed other notions of dying in community which are more meaningful in contemporary society. Seale (1995) uses the accounts of relatives of people who died alone to argue that society is very concerned to maintain the idea that people die belonging to a community which accommodates the deaths of its members in an orderly fashion. Hence, the body which lies undiscovered within a shared social space is shocking even to strangers.

Contemporary rituals and spiritualities

The notion of privatised death is usually linked to the decline in, or absence of, public ceremony and shared social ritual. Although Walter has argued that contemporary Britons are very insecure about the appropriateness of social rituals (Walter, 1994; Walter et al, 1995) there is growing evidence in emerging funeral and disposal practices that 'postmodern death' has caught up on the use of ritual and translated traditional, formally structured expressions into more fluid, individually customised mechanisms (see Chapter Seven). Psychologically based therapeutic interventions have also been quick to transport the essence of ritual into their therapies (Grainger, 1998), offering a framework within which a customised ritual, meaningful for the individual and family, may be shaped. Lay people, too, according to Williams, ritualise for themselves their experiences of dying and bereavement, selecting and interweaving from different traditions and cultural influences (Williams, 1990). Embedded in the search for, or confirmation of, a satisfactory philosophical framework for the respondents in my study was the establishment, or reinforcement, of individual rituals which were personally meaningful. One man, although an atheist, described this process in quasi-religious terms:

> ... you've got to try to take whatever you can from that (and I don't just mean on an individual basis) and then distribute it ... It's a peculiar mix of getting on with it but also thinking about others who perhaps will never impinge on your life, and, technically, it is almost a sort of religious attitude. (Lloyd, 1996, p 305)

When these processes are represented in concrete form, they illustrate what, in an increasing crossover of disciplinary approaches to exploring death, sociologists have begun to refer to as the 'embodiment of emotion' and anthropologists as the 'emotion of material culture' (see Tarlow, 1999, for an account of the missed dimension of the emotions of bereavement in work on the archaeology of memorials).

Walter debates whether the rise in New Age practices around death reflects a resurgence in religious approaches to death or simply a search for alternative forms of ritual to mark it. He concludes that it is in fact both: a reaction against the medicalising and technicising of death and a re-spiritualisation of death (Walter, 1993). Walter also points out that New Age spiritualities are self-actualising and thus bring the focus back to 'my own death' from concentration on death of 'the other' which the modern funeral and grief counselling industries have combined to produce (see Chapter Seven for a discussion of 'alternative' funerals). Meanwhile, the broader question of contemporary expressions of religion and spirituality belongs both to the revision of modern death and to discussion of end-of-life care (Chapter Five). It is no longer sufficient to conclude that contemporary death is secularised when the evidence of religious and cultural pluralism coexisting with scientific advances raises important questions for the management of dying and bereavement.

Attitudes and beliefs about death

So far we have been looking at analyses of death driven by sociologists and anthropologists, which take as their starting point the way in which societies organise themselves to accommodate the processes of death, and the juxtaposition of the continuing community of the living with those who are dying or have died in living memory. The phrase 'passed away', far from being just a euphemism for death employed by individuals to avoid its harsh reality, is, in fact, redolent with social meaning.

An alternative approach from psychology, philosophy and theology is concerned with the challenge to human existence of the fact of death. This can be at the level of the individual or shared humanity. Feifel (1959) reminds us that human beings are distinguished among life forms by the knowledge that they will die, and by their ability to reflect on that fact across their individual and communal dimensions.

Psychological approaches

Although the latest of these three disciplines to engage with the study of death, psychology has taken over the field when it comes to theorising bereavement and grief (which are discussed in Chapter Four). The emphasis on psychopathology and psychiatric interventions can be seen as a direct outworking of its preoccupation with fear of death, and anxiety and denial in the face of death. These attitudes are examined within the broader approach of *constructs* of death, attitudes being categorised as positive, negative or neutral psychological states. These studies have emanated largely from the US, following Feifel's pioneering work. The earlier studies variously measured death awareness, fear and anxiety in relation to age, personality type and religiosity variables. In general, people were reported to be more aware and accepting of death in old age. However, Fortner and Neimeyer (1999) revisited these earlier studies, and concluded that four factors contributed to heightened death anxiety in older populations: physical health problems, a history of psychological distress, weaker religious beliefs, and reduced life satisfaction or personal resilience. This finding is particularly significant given the contemporary picture of old age, with people living longer but with more health problems and disabilities, including the prevalence of a range of degenerative conditions, and with evidence that dying in old age is in many ways the most 'disadvantaged dying'. Fortner and Neimeyer also found that older people in institutional care displayed greater fear of death than those living at home. Moreover, evidence that fear of death remains stable in old age is based on studies of 65- to 75-year-olds; we know remarkably little about death anxiety among the oldest groups (Cicirelli, 2001). Chapter Five examines these issues in depth.

Three lines of enquiry have been pursued in some depth: the relationship between ill-health, particularly terminal illness, and death anxiety; the relationship between religiosity and attitudes to death; and the impact of their own attitudes towards death on care-giving among health professionals. These findings from earlier and recent work are helpfully presented in an overview of psychological research on death attitudes provided by Neimeyer and colleagues (Neimeyer et al, 2004). The picture is both complex and contradictory, but the following central points are worth highlighting:

- Whether or not people who are terminally ill display high death anxiety levels appears to depend on the relationship between their health and other variables, rather than the proximity of death per se.

- Although psychology originally viewed religion as the source of much anxiety, a growing body of work suggests that religious and spiritual beliefs promote acceptance of death.
- Professional care-givers who themselves display anxious or avoidant attitudes towards death are more likely to hold negative views about ageing and to act conservatively (for example resisting making a terminal diagnosis or giving palliative care).

Psychological interest in attitudes to death has seen something of a resurgence in late modernity. It differs from earlier work in that it is stimulated by significant sociopolitical events and contexts. Thus both the AIDS pandemic and 9/11 have been investigated as situations creating heightened death anxiety, related not so much to individual variables but observable among particular social groups and across whole communities (Neimeyer et al, 2004). Nevertheless, the psychologists concern themselves with the factors creating individual variation – such as greater fear of death among HIV-positive gay men who lacked family support. There is a similar interest in the impact of religiosity. Notable about this contemporary research into the relationship between sociopolitical context and death attitudes is its narrow frame of reference. The AIDS pandemic, for example, is confined to the North American gay population – similar studies in South Africa might throw up quite different measures of significance. The impact of 9/11 does not look at death anxiety among Muslim populations, despite the acknowledged threat to the personal safety and well-being of a whole sector of the population as the targets of jingoistic pronouncements and violent outbursts.

Approaches from theology and philosophy

I am considering the contributions from these two disciplines together because, in what has to be only a brief incursion into the huge amount of material which they have generated around death, they share a core approach: the attempt to conceptualise death. Moreover, their conceptual positions are remarkably similar; it is in the response made to the intellectual position that the differences emerge. These concepts and constructs of death have to be translated into working models if they are to assist us in understanding our responses to death. Although this work is rich in theorising, it is the one field in the study of death which has generated as yet few empirical studies, and therefore I am drawing substantially on my own work, which has explored spiritual and philosophical issues in death, dying and bereavement through both a study of the literature and empirical work (Lloyd, 1995, 1996, 1997) and has subsequently developed this material to explore the notion of transcultural spirituality (Holloway, 2006a). The common feature of the varied people in my study, independent of the holding of defined religious belief, was that they recognised at some level that they were engaged in an ontological quest (Lloyd, 1996). This was also identified by the secular professionals as one of the distinguishing features of working with people who are dying or bereaved (Lloyd, 1997).

An overview analysis of the literature[3] reveals a number of recurring and interrelated themes. Some are obviously complementary, others represent opposing positions, and others appear at different points on a continuum. Table 3.1 summarises each position.

Table 3.1: Typology of concepts of death

Concept	Meaning
Death as light	*In death is achieved ultimate fulfilment, it is essentially the consummation of the life.*
Death as darkness	*Death destroys the meaning in life; tragedy and suffering are senseless.*
Death as mystery	*We cannot fully understand death.*
Death as end	*Death must be simply and pragmatically accepted.*
Death as transition	*Death is a stage which moves our existence on.*
Death as limit	*Death should be seen as a boundary which bestows meaning on life.*
Death as borderline situation	*Death pushes us to the limits of personal resources in which ultimate freedom may be achieved.*
Death as the only truly personal act	*In dying we exercise ultimate freedom.*
Death as passivity	*We accept our own experience of death.*
Death and life together make sense	*Each must be examined and understood in relation to the other.*
Death as natural event	*Mortality is the natural condition of human existence.*
Death as unnatural event	*Death is sometimes violent and premature.*
Death as hope	*In death is healing and release.*

At first sight these positions may seem impenetrable to the non-specialist reader, or of no practical application to the practitioner. However, we can start to make connections with familiar themes in the experiences of dying and bereavement as we consider them further.

Three broad groupings emerge across these thirteen positions, which take either a positive or negative view of death, or a dialectical approach.

The positive view of death

The work of the German philosopher, Martin Heidegger, is often taken as the starting point for proponents of largely positive approaches to conceptualising death, although Heidegger himself can be understood quite differently: Macquarrie suggests that Heidegger helps us to understand how death strips away all illusions from life but leaves us with nothing with which to face the cold fact of death (Macquarrie, 1973). Heidegger explored what it means to be human, to be mortal, suggesting that only because of the possibility of 'not being' can 'being' be defined, and the potential within human existence be realised (Heidegger, 1962). Heidegger describes human existence as lived out in the knowledge, or 'anxiety', of our death, which is not the same as the fear of death which has preoccupied psychology (Edgar, 1996). According to Heidegger, we may live our lives inauthentically, that is, avoiding and evading the implications of mortality, or authentically, that is, accepting the fact of death as a prerequisite to fulfilling our potential. One woman in my research explained her 42-year-old husband's struggle to 'live his dying' authentically:

> 'There was a sense in which it was the end of his natural lifespan … a sense of looking at the richness of what had been achieved … it was important for him to make sense of "God" before because he didn't expect anything coming beyond.' (Lloyd, 1996, p. 302)

In the sense that the closer we actually come to death, the greater the potential for it to bestow meaning on life, Heidegger describes life as advancing towards death. A similar orientation is reflected in Jung's notion of life curving up to its mid-point and down towards death with equal intensity (Jung, 1959). Rahner sees death as life's 'consummation' (Rahner, 1963). This notion of achieving potential, even personal growth, through facing death has been popularised among the counselling community through the work of Elizabeth Kubler-Ross (Kubler-Ross, 1975). The following quotes from three women give their own versions of the same theme:

> 'This has opened doors to experience that I wouldn't have had access to.' (Lloyd, 1996, p 303)
>
> 'I appreciate life no matter how low the quality.' (Lloyd, 1996, p 305)
>
> 'I think bad things happen to make room for the good.' (Lloyd, 1996, p 306)

Plato's argument that only in death can the soul achieve true freedom is built upon in various ways to explore the freedom which is achieved in death. At first sight this idea seems deeply inimical to the contemporary mind, more used to modern medicine's struggle to wrest control from death. Jaspers sees human existence as a constant encounter with 'borderline situations' where one is brought to the limits of personal resources; the realisation of death as the ultimate borderline provides freedom and release from the struggle (Jaspers, 1967). Others take this notion further by arguing that in giving oneself to death, the individual achieves the ultimate assertion of the self, free from other considerations (Boros, 1973). Palliative care workers will recognise here the patient who decides that they just want to be 'made comfortable', or who dies when their relative leaves the room just for a moment. One of my respondents phrased it thus: 'I deign to die' (Lloyd, 1996, p 304).

Finally, death, somewhat paradoxically, can be turned into hope. Most usually in theological literature this is pursued in the specific beliefs of redemption and resurrection. However, such concepts are also presented in terms of the implications of individual lives and how they are lived, for continuing human existence (Kung, 1984; Moltman, 1989). This is not unlike Young and Cullen's comments from their study of death in East London, that death contains the potential to regenerate morality and human solidarity, that in stripping away the 'trappings' of life, it enables individuals and communities to focus on the essentials of human existence (Young and Cullen, 1996). One of my respondents, although not a person of religious faith, explained how she had made sense of the death of her baby: 'He gave up his life to make me take up a new life' (Lloyd, 1996, p 302).

The current trend towards funeral services serving as celebrations of the life which has gone might also be seen as a search to find hope within death. So, too, might the general sense of trying to achieve something positive out of an otherwise very dark experience:[4] 'I had nothing else to cling onto belief-wise ... this feeling of turning it into the positives' (Lloyd, 1996, p 305).

The negative view of death

The most extreme statement of the negativity of death comes from Jean-Paul Sartre, who declares that death sweeps away meaning from life, destroying all life's possibilities. From this perspective, tragedy is meaningless suffering. Developing the work of Freud, Feuerbach sees religion, and particularly belief in eternal life, as a psychological projection used to deal with the threat of extinction. The only response, he argues, must be to orientate oneself towards the here-and-now and accept that in death we are swallowed up in nothingness (Feuerbach, 1957). The challenge of death to life's meanings is serious and represents a threat which may lie behind the ostracism from former friends often experienced by bereaved people. The anguish of despair also engenders a helplessness in professional carers which is particularly difficult for them to deal with. This is perhaps why very few people assert the position of meaninglessness in the face of suffering. We shall see in the following chapter how 'meaning-making' is becoming one of the dominant approaches to understanding and intervening in grief. Ministers of religion will be particularly familiar with the discomfort of being confronted with questions such as this woman presents after the death of her child on the operating table: 'My life had just been completely shattered, but why? ... surely it can't be pointless ... it's not for nothing' (Lloyd, 1996, p 301).

The negative view of death would say that it is. This approach to death confronts the existential pain of death head on and refuses to offer any comfort, including in religion (Collopy, 1978). This is in contrast to the essentially positive approach, which does not deny the destruction of death but sees a positive approach to dying as the way through its darkness (Linnane, 2001).

The dialectical approach

The third approach can be seen to emerge more directly from human experience, in that it struggles with both the light and the darkness of death. As we have seen from the few quotations given above, ordinary people articulate both sides of the coin when death becomes of immediate personal concern. It is also a feature of all the world religions that there is a long tradition of addressing suffering but within a framework of hope (Holloway, 2006a). This is in contrast to philosophy where the 'problem' of death was traditionally deemed the 'philosopher's touchstone' and, some argue, overwhelming. In current philosophical research, themes of happiness and well-being have replaced death. The development of secularised rituals around death also stumble on this point, as Ros Coward, writing about secular funerals, highlights:

> The modern need for consolation and celebration abandons the harshness of traditional rituals that can be infinitely more cathartic. (Coward, 2002)

Three sub-themes are used to hold together the two sides of death:

- death as paradox
- death as mystery
- death as the stimulator of life's deepest responses.

Taken together, these explore the idea that only through grappling with death do we take away the fear of death; the concept is not one of removing the darkness, however, but of illuminating the darkness, of 'looking the negative in the face' (Jungel, 1975, p 53). Paradoxically, as we seek to understand life, we find ourselves trying to find answers to the dilemmas created for life in death (Jungel, 1975). Yet it remains a mystery, evoking some of our deepest responses about the human condition which connect past, present and future generations (Tillich, 1959). Sheila Cassidy,[5] a hospice doctor, describes how this approach finds expression for her in the world of modern medicine:

> Slowly, as the years go by, I learn about the importance of powerlessness. I experience it in my own life and I live with it in my work. The secret is not to be afraid of it – not to run away. The dying know we are not God … All they ask is that we do not desert them. (Cassidy, 1988, p 64)

It is empowerment, rather than powerlessness, however, which is the objective of contemporary health and social care. In Chapter Eight we consider how these two concepts may come together in practice with people who are dying and bereaved. The following quotations suggest different ways in which my respondents were trying to deal with the ambiguities around life and death in their own experience:

> 'I realised that the operation could make death come quicker, on the other hand, if I was meant to stay here then, yes, I will do … I don't go to meet it, but …' (Lloyd, 1996, p 304)
>
> 'There are no set answers and there are no answers written down in a book … I've just had to make a whole of all the bits and pieces.' (Lloyd, 1996, p 304)
>
> 'Because of the nature of the disease, it was just one of those things … if you're good, kind, thoughtful and generous it can happen to you just as it can happen to anyone else.' (Lloyd, 1996, p 305)
>
> 'I've seen a lot of suffering … I've consoled others so I must console myself.' (Lloyd, 1996, p 303)

Jackson (1982) suggests that the function of religion is to provide the basis for a philosophy of life and death which sustains the highest spiritual aspirations in life, yet has a realistic acceptance of death. We can make that more inclusive by suggesting that the insights of religion may facilitate the development of a philosophy of life and death for the individual which enables them to approach death with wholeness. Both Peter Kostenbaum and I have suggested some everyday translations in the conceptualising of death. Kostenbaum suggests that philosophies of death can be seen in the values by which the ordinary person seeks to conduct their life (Table 3.2).

Table 3.2: Kostenbaum's values by which people live

1	*We need death in order to savour life.*
2	*Death is an 'invention' needed and created for the sake of feeling alive.*
3	*Death puts us in touch with the sense of an individual experience.*
4	*Death makes possible decisions for authenticity – courage and integrity.*
5	*Death gives us the strength to make major decisions.*
6	*Death reveals the importance of intimacy in life.*
7	*Death helps us ascribe meaning to our lives retroactively.*
8	*Death shows us the importance of ego-transcending achievements.*
9	*Death shows us the path to self-esteem and gives us the capacity to do something important.*

I have translated my typology into a number of common expressions which will be recognised by those familiar with death or with working with people who are dying or bereaved (Table 3.3).

It will not have escaped the reader that there is no recent literature cited in the discussion of the conceptualisation of death in philosophy and theology. Like social science, philosophy and theology in late modernity appear to be rather more interested in a mosaic of themes rather than the grand design and there is no recent systematic study of death on which to draw. In fact, much of the more recent work which deals directly with beliefs around death has come from other disciplines. Two areas of interest should be noted: interest in an 'afterlife'

Table 3.3: Contemporary stances on death

Traditional concept	Contemporary translation
Death as light	*'I've grown through this.'*
Death as darkness	*'It's such a waste, it doesn't make sense.'*
Death as mystery	*'I just go with the flow now.'*
Death as end	*'That's it, no sense worrying about it.'*
Death as transition	*'It wasn't really him lying there, only his body.'*
Death as limit	*'It concentrates the mind, makes you realise what's important.'*
Death as borderline situation	*'I've reached my limit.'* *'There's no going back now.'*
Death as the only truly personal act	*'I've got to do this one on my own.'*
Death as passivity	*'It comes to us all.'*
Death and life together make sense	*'If you didn't have death, you wouldn't have life.'*
Death as natural event	*'She was ready to go, it was like her time had come.'*
Death as unnatural event	*'He was snatched away, snuffed out.'*
Death as hope	*'He's at peace now.'* *'I'm going home.'*

and psychical research into phenomena such as 'near-death experiences' (which became Elizabeth Kubler-Ross's consuming interest); and an interest in spiritual bonds alongside the development of continuing bonds theory in bereavement research (Klass and Goss, 1999), which is discussed in the next chapter. The continuing bonds theorists are more concerned with the sociopolitical functions that retaining such bonds exert in different cultures and historical periods than with the intrinsic beliefs. Similarly, although there is recent work reiterating belief in some form of continuing existence in all the major religions (Haddow, 2002) it is left to New Age devotees to pursue visions of an afterlife. The current preoccupations of the main religions and theology are with the ethical issues arising from end-of-life care and the dimension of spiritual care.

Dying

The study of dying brings in contributors from all disciplines, but with a more applied angle in terms of the implications for care and carers. The earliest theorising was developed from observational studies of care of people who were dying. Glaser and Strauss (1965 and 1967) focused the lens of social interactionism on ward life in American hospitals, an approach replicated by the British sociologist, David Field, in his study of nurses' and doctors' behaviour towards people on cancer wards (Field, 1989). Hinton's study of dying is another classic (Hinton, 1967 and 1980), which, in its vivid portrayal of the emotional pain and isolation of the dying person, contributed significantly to the picture of modern death.

Awareness contexts

Glaser and Strauss identified four 'awareness contexts': *closed awareness*, where everyone but the patient knows or deduces that s/he is dying; *suspected awareness*, where the patient has not been told (though others have) and tries to confirm her/his suspicions; *mutual pretence awareness*, where the different parties (patient, relatives, staff) know or decide that the person is dying but keep up a mutual pretence that the other person is unaware; and *open awareness*, where everyone knows and openly acts or communicates on that basis.

The issue and practice of disclosure of a terminal diagnosis have generated considerable research and continue to be debated, despite a broad consensus that individuals who wish to know should be told. Field summarised the position over a decade ago, and more recent work suggests that, at core, the issues have not changed:

- The fact that they are terminally ill is often concealed from patients in British hospitals even now (the current debate focuses more on communication problems with older patients and lack of a clear-cut terminal condition even though they are evidently in the 'dying phase' of life – see Chapter Five for further discussion).
- The main reasons for this avoidance have to do with protecting the patient from depression and anxiety and staff from the disruption to their normal routines of becoming too closely involved in the emotional and psychological problems of dying (the growth in palliative care wards and hospice provision over the past decade undoubtedly provides a counter-position, but there are considerable inequalities in access to this provision and some suggestions – see earlier discussion – that hospice staff also avoid the actual subject of death).
- The evidence points towards most people becoming aware that they are dying even if they are not actually told (the current position is probably that 'disclosure' is wrapped up in ongoing discussion of treatment options and decisions).
- Substantial numbers of people when asked indicate that they would want to know if they are dying (the current debate is also linked to euthanasia and physician-assisted suicide).
- Those who do not wish to know seem not to 'hear' or to reinterpret the information (my own research [Lloyd, 1997] demonstrated that even where professionals claimed to have had open discussion with the patient of the fact that they were dying, a number of patients had not interpreted having a terminal diagnosis to mean that they were dying).
- There are strong moral and ethical reasons for disclosure, arising from evidence that secrecy and suspicion heighten anxiety, distress and loneliness, and non-disclosure denies people the opportunity to put their affairs in order and to face death together as a family (these ethical and moral imperatives remain but are complicated by the power to prolong life, or end life, brought about by significant treatment developments – see Chapter Five).

- There is a growing consensus that 'open awareness' eases the stress for patients, families and staff, but when and how to disclose remains problematic (some features of the contemporary context of health and social care militate against good practice but other initiatives such as 'dying pathways' are facilitative – see Chapters Two and Five).

Open communication

In contemporary healthcare there is broad consensus that sharing the diagnosis eases the stress for all concerned and may be the key to empowering the dying person (Sheldon, 1997) but there is continuing unease about the practice of communicating 'bad news' and the moral and ethical dilemmas surrounding the management of the knowledge of dying. Twycross (1997) is particularly concerned with the doctor's dilemma that to destroy hope is to destroy the essential person; Timmermans (2005) argues that in keeping a poor prognosis from the patient, doctors continue to attribute to themselves the power to maintain or destroy life. This is one area where secular professionals might draw on pastoral theology, which has paid considerable attention to the concept and practice of hope (Boney, 1975). Rumbold has particularly examined the application of theological insights in palliative care (Rumbold, 1986 and 2002). He defines 'hope' thus:

> Hope is not the same thing as wishful thinking or unfounded optimism, nor is it merely a set of concepts to be given intellectual assent. Rather, hope has its birth in a realistic assessment of our situation, and is grounded in our experiences and the values by which we live. (Rumbold, 1986, p 59)

Rumbold suggests that people possess hope along a continuum, whereby at one end the dying person (and presumably those closely surrounding them, including caring professionals) is able to affirm creative possibilities in the face of death and at the other is resigned to despair. The process of striving towards 'mature hope' is one which he suggests the individual must undertake for themselves. This definition of hope cannot be 'given' to a person but does not preclude the possibility of a shared journey (Lloyd, 1995). The respondents in my own study who suggested that cancer rather than death was discussed in the hospice further implied that no one facilitated their reflection on their own dying and imminent death (Lloyd, 1996 and 1997).

Despite continuing ambivalence and ambiguity about disclosure of the diagnosis, Seale and Cartwright present evidence that practice changed significantly in the direction of open communication between 1969 and 1987 (Seale and Cartwright, 1994). However, they also suggest a number of caveats:

- Professionals preferred to give the news to relatives, rather than to the patient her/himself.

- People who knew that they were dying were more likely to have guessed this than to have been told.
- Both relatives and patients were more likely to be told what the problem was than that the condition would lead to death.
- When asked to reflect on whether the state of awareness in which their relative died was 'for the best', a majority of bereaved people stated that it was, implying that some people would not have wanted to know that they were dying (although the researchers do acknowledge the limitations of allowing the views of bereaved relatives to speak for the dying person in retrospect).

Dying trajectories

The process of dying is the other main thrust in theorising dying. Glaser and Strauss followed the anthropological work on rites of passage in conceptualising dying as 'status passage' which is jointly negotiated by the patient, family and professional carers. However, when death is sudden and unexpected, there is no time or opportunity to negotiate this passage and significant social and psychological disruption occurs. Glaser and Strauss identified two main trajectories – that is, how long the person is expected to live and the anticipated pattern of care – *quick dying* and *slow dying*. Within each of the two trajectories there is both expected and unexpected death. For example, a person who is terminally ill may linger longer than expected or die suddenly at a point which is not expected clinically. Even the expected pattern could be problematic – the patient dying at a shift changeover, or emergency routines being operationalised when the relatives had briefly left the ward, for example. The important point to highlight here is that it was the tensions created between medical and ward procedures and the needs of patients and relatives, particularly where either of these was at odds with the timescale of actual events, which proved problematic.

This raises a number of issues for contemporary healthcare, given that the moves towards 'best practice' are commonly in the direction of identifying a care pathway with predetermined options for procedures and decision making. Timmermans (2005) provides an interesting update on dying trajectories set into the contemporary context of 'managed dying'. Using the term 'death brokering' he analyses how medical professionals continue to control dying but infuse their practice with the values of patient-centred care and the 'good death'. This contemporary context for dying is explored fully in Chapter Five, but here it is useful to note that the professionally determined trajectory may not be disrupted without severe disturbance to the ethos of care. So, for example, a patient in the hospice may be palliatively sedated but requests to hasten death cause discomfort; relatives are encouraged to say their goodbyes when staff decide the time has come. Costello's recent work on nursing dying patients in hospital found nurses expressing the same tensions about patients dying unexpectedly or inconveniently as had been highlighted in the 1960s by Glaser and Strauss (Costello, 2001, 2006).

Stages of dying

The second influential approach, particularly for practitioners, has been Elizabeth Kubler-Ross's stages of dying (Kubler-Ross, 1970). It is now commonplace for 'stage theory', as it came to be known, to be criticised as overly prescriptive, generalising from subjective data and failing to recognise the range of individual variation. However, Kubler-Ross's theory, generated from her observations as a psychiatrist of terminally ill patients in a Chicago hospital, has been one of the most widely applied with an enduring popularity with trainers in grief counselling. Kubler-Ross claimed that people who know that they are dying pass through five stages in linear fashion: *denial*, *anger*, *bargaining*, *depression*, until finally reaching *acceptance*. This is essentially a psychological process and emotional response, without attention to either social context (although she does link denial to isolation) or philosophical underpinnings (although in her later life Kubler-Ross became obsessed with near-death experiences as psychic phenomena with spiritual overtones). The processes which she described continue to be identified by theorists, but it is the deterministic fashion in which her stages have been applied to all experiences of loss and the conflation of Kubler-Ross's work with other work on the process of grief and mourning under the umbrella of stage theory (see Chapter Four), which has led to the greatest criticism.

Religiosity, spirituality and terminal illness

Palliative care has, historically, worked on the general assumption that a spiritual dimension becomes important when people are dying. The hospice philosophy contained spiritual care in its mission from the outset, and one of the criticisms made of the earliest hospices during the height of the AIDS crisis was that their overtly (Christian) religious ethos acted to exclude many people. The relationship between belief and how people cope with terminal illness is of considerable interest to researchers, although this body of work is scant by comparison with much else in the theorising of death, and the evidence on a number of points remains ambiguous and contested. Some key points which have emerged so far in what continues to be an area requiring much further investigation are:

- A beneficial effect on health and well-being of religious activity (Koenig et al, 1998), and of spiritual beliefs (Walsh et al, 2002) is claimed, but levels and types of religiosity are known to be significantly different in the US from the UK and northern Europe, and evidence about the relationships between religious belief, spiritual well-being and health status remains ambiguous (for example, James and Wells, 2002; McClain et al, 2003; McGrath, 2003).
- Serious illness may present a crisis of faith for some people (Lloyd, 1996) and weak belief is associated with depression (Charlton et al, 2005).
- The main world religions are in agreement that individuals become more concerned with transcendental issues as they age (Thursby, 1992; Howse,

2004) but there is speculation that the 'baby-boomer' generation (those born in the population increase after the Second World War, credited with creating the culture of the 1960s) may alter this perspective as they resist the ageing process.
- There is little understanding of spiritual need among people who are dying, and professionals are often unsure of the meaning of spiritual care in practice (Lloyd, 1995; Cobb, 2001); despite the proliferation of standardised spirituality scales, few have been devised from, or tested on, either terminally ill or older populations.

The concentration from the pastoral theology and pastoral care literature has been on offering spiritual care, rather than on developing theoretical insights into the spiritual needs of the dying person. In fact, the pastoral counselling movement has itself become profoundly secularised resulting, Dawe argues, in it losing touch with its own religious, spiritual and intellectual resources (Dawe, 1975). A small amount of work has examined spiritual pain. In a UK-wide questionnaire survey I conducted with hospital chaplaincies and social work departments, 86 per cent said that they recognised spiritual pain in dying and bereaved people. Understanding of spiritual pain draws, on the one hand, on spiritual traditions, which suggest that the path to spiritual growth is through suffering, to, on the other hand, more modern interpretations, which suggest that profound discomfort occurs when the inner self feels alienation, dissonance or deep conflict (Burton, 2004). Heyse-Moore argues that this is common to all people of all beliefs, and can be recognised in physical and psychological symptoms and relationship problems, as well as those more obvious features of existential anguish such as desolation and a profound sense of meaninglessness (Heyse-Moore, 1996).

Conclusion

The search for a richly textured, theoretically sophisticated understanding of death and dying goes on. This chapter has considered how some of the earliest anthropological work on ritual and symbolism continues to have relevance as societies in the developed world gradually replace the traditional ways of dealing with death and dying. In seeking to chart and understand new practices, there is much that can be learnt from the patterns and meanings established in more primitive or earlier societies. What appears to endure is the need for ritual, albeit in our society individualised and personalised customs and symbols may become the norm as fewer people adhere to established belief systems. Yet there is tentative evidence that people look for social validation of their individual rites, and continue to be concerned that dying takes place in community and is marked by the community. The sociological study of death, which demonstrated how modern societies distanced themselves from death, established the importance of understanding death as a social phenomenon, but there are good reasons for us now to question some of the pictures which it painted.

Theories of dying remain largely unrevised. Possibly the main reason for this is that a significant deficit in the research is the construction of narratives about death and dying from the first-hand accounts of people who are terminally ill (Clark and Seymour, 1999). Such evidence as we have is located in a few small-scale studies, which does not as yet constitute a substantial body of work where new theories can be seen to emerge. There are, however, growing trends, for example, the interest in spirituality. Perhaps the indications are that the study of dying, in tune with postmodernism, is not looking for overarching theories. It is particularly concerned, however, with the ethical and practical issues of end-of-life care, which we look at in Chapter Five.

As we pay more attention to the relationship between the individual experience and social representation of death, there is a need to integrate accounts of individual attitudes towards death with its management in society. Psychology has contributed a vast body of work on the impact of individuals' attitudes to death on their behaviours, including the behaviour of those in the caring professions. Yet without social and cultural contextualisation, it is hard to make sense of this information. The attitudes held by older people are a case in point, with particular implications for the development of appropriate end-of-life care in the contemporary context.

Morever, there is much still to be explored about the beliefs around death held by people in late modernity and how these impact on the way we manage both the process of dying and the death. It may be generally recognised that death presents an existential challenge corporately and often an existential crisis for the individual, but there has been little exploration of changing beliefs and spiritual practices around death in contemporary society. Failure to attend to the framework of belief surrounding death and dying leaves us, arguably, dangerously adrift in the ethics of end-of-life decision making and the management of the psychosocial realities of dying. The changing identity of the dying person as he or she moves towards death is an angle often forgotten in discussions about end-of-life technologies, although the hospice movement continues to remind us of their personhood.

The theoretical approaches to death and dying reviewed in this chapter have for too long been pursued in disciplinary isolation. If we are to develop an understanding of death and dying which meets the considerable challenges of late modernity, we must engage in a genuine interdisciplinary encounter. Only such an approach will assist in the social, psychological and philosophical negotiations in which we as societies and individuals engage as we attempt to accommodate death and dying.

Key questions for practitioners

1. Which theories and approaches to death and dying do I feel most comfortable with? What do they contribute to my practice?
2. Are there any with which I am uncomfortable? Why? What, if anything, could I take from these which might enhance my practice?
3. What issues are most challenging for me around death and dying? Personally? In my work? What could the theorising of death and dying contribute to helping me deal with these issues?
4. What do I see as the continuing gaps? In the theories? In my own work?

Notes

[1] CRUSE is a national bereavement support network in the UK.

[2] Excerpt from 'Aubade', Philip Larkin.

[3] The literature considered was from Christian theology and western philosophy. However, I am indebted to my colleagues from the Spirituality seminar of the 2005 meeting of the International Work Group on Death, Dying and Bereavement for their application of these concepts in the light of their different religious and cultural backgrounds.

[4] I am grateful to my colleague Dr Julian Stern for his amendment of my original articulation of this theme to encompass the secular vision of hope in death.

[5] Sheila Cassidy first came to public attention when she was imprisoned and tortured by the military Junta for treating a wounded revolutionary whilst working as a doctor in Chile in the 1970s.

FOUR

Understanding bereavement and grief

Introduction

The sociological study of death which began in the mid-twentieth century spawned what for a long time was the dominant area of academic interest – the study of grief. Geoffrey Gorer's classic work on death in modern Britain took as its starting point the observation that the restriction of public mourning and reduction in ritual which had come about in post-war Britain had deprived individuals of support in their grieving, and, moreover, created an atmosphere in which mourning was treated as 'a weakness, a self-indulgence, a reprehensible bad habit, instead of as a psychological necessity' (Gorer, 1965, p 113). In the death-denying societies of the mid-twentieth century, grief as a problematic phenomenon began to be theorised and interventions developed and refined on that basis. In fact, long before 'modern death' was discovered, Freud had been interested in the importance for psychoanalysis of loss of a love object, and the intra-psychic processes set in motion by significant loss. Thus, right from the start, attempts to better understand grief went hand-in-hand with attempts to help those whose grief looked problematic.

Guidance of those professionals who care for people who are dying and bereaved continues to be one of the chief stimulators of the study of bereavement. Yet the application of theoretical underpinnings has not been unproblematic and much of the more recent revision is concerned with the assertion of lay experience of bereavement over the professional discourse on grief. Tony Walter, using the term 'policing grief', looks at the many ways in which the over-regulated use of models of grief by professionals has led to dissonance between their attempts to help and the actual and varied experiences of bereaved people (Walter, 1999). On the other side of the coin, it has often been practitioners who have pointed out the inappropriateness of 'one size fits all', or over-prescriptive, models to the diverse encounters with death and dying which they meet in their work. There is also some merit in the claim that much of the problem with bereavement counselling which Walter points to has arisen outside of the professional sphere, through overzealous application of reductionist models by volunteer bereavement counsellors. To counter that claim, one of the oldest and largest bereavement support agencies in the UK – CRUSE – maintains that their counsellors are trained to discover from the bereaved themselves how to understand their personal experience of grief (Arnason and Hafsteinsson, 2003).

Before we turn to the theories of grief, it is perhaps useful to define some of the terms used and the ways in which they are used. I have already mentioned 'bereavement', 'mourning' and 'grief', and the reader may be forgiven for thinking that these terms may be used interchangeably. It is important to establish their precise meanings, because they reflect different aspects of this experience of losing a person with whom one has had a significant relationship:

- *Bereavement* is the experience of loss occasioned by death. Some analysts do apply the term to any experience of loss, but its technical meaning applies only to loss through death.[1] However, other losses of a significant person, for example through divorce, may feel like a bereavement. Aside from the issue of the significance of the loss, the use of the term 'bereavement' relating to loss of a person through death, or similar circumstance, implies a social and philosophical context which is absent from other losses such as loss of a limb; moreover, such losses are defined by the individual experience, whereas widowhood, for example, is a universally defined social state.
- *Mourning* is the pattern of behaviour engaged in by those who are bereaved, and the term carries with it the connotation that this behaviour is to a greater or lesser extent socially defined and publicly recognised. Thus, all funeral attendees, as well as those most closely bereaved, may be referred to as the 'mourners', and in some cultures 'professional mourners' are employed.
- *Grief* and *grieving* are descriptions of the individual's psychological and emotional responses to loss, 'grief' being the descriptor applied to the state and 'grieving' implying the processes which the person experiences and psychological and emotional strategies which they may employ. These are commonly manifested in certain outward behaviours. The grief experienced following a loss other than of a person through death may be entirely analogous to the grief which follows a bereavement, because grief is determined by what the lost 'object' represented to the grieving person. It is because this does not always accord with the assumptions of others, that the individual's grief may be misconstrued or not recognised.

Thus, although there are clear distinctions in the meanings attached to the terms 'bereavement', 'mourning' and 'grief', and attempting to separate those out underlines the complexity of grief, there is, of course, considerable overlap in their usage because they remain, to a significant degree, entangled in the individual experience of bereavement. In a recent analysis of grief entitled 'Mourning and Memory', Robert Neimeyer and colleagues discuss how grief as a response to loss is 'situated' sociologically, psychologically and psychiatrically (Neimeyer et al, 2002). Grief is a complex phenomenon which presents the individual with psychological, sociological and emotional challenges. It is also an experience which is socially constructed and must be accommodated in society. Moreover, it presents the individual, and sometimes the wider community, with existential and spiritual challenges (Lloyd, 1996 and 1997), but this dimension continues to be peculiarly lacking in current attempts to integrate disciplinary perspectives. In all other respects, more recent work on grief has been marked by theoretical diversity (Stroebe, 2001). However, it is from psychology and psychiatry that the most sustained attempts to explain and understand grief continue to emanate.

Attachment and loss

Central to the early work on grief, and of continuing importance in current discussions, is an understanding of the attachments which human beings form to a 'love' object. The word 'love' here implies the full spectrum from the physical attachment formed with the source of early succour, to a deeply held emotional commitment to another adult. John Bowlby's work on attachment, separation and loss (Bowlby, 1969, 1973 and 1980), developed initially from his study of the effects on young children of being deprived of their mother, has been extraordinarily influential in the development of frameworks for childcare practice, but has also formed the basis for theorising grief in adults. Bowlby described a process in which the young child forms a primary bond with the natural mother (although his later work acknowledged that the primary attachment object is not always the mother and other revisions emphasise that multiple significant bonds may be formed). Bowlby drew on work from biology to liken this process in humans to the way in which the newborn in many animal species become fixated on the first available object (known as 'imprinting').

For the purposes of this brief summary, it is the nature of the attachments formed, and the impact of losing them, which have most influenced the subsequent work on grief based on attachment theory. The work of the British psychiatrist, Colin Murray Parkes, combines research and clinical work on the making and breaking of attachments and their impact on bereavement, as the theoretical basis for therapeutic treatment (Parkes, 2006). As Parkes summarises, Bowlby and two associated researchers, Mary Ainsworth and Mary Maine, identified these early attachments as 'secure' or 'insecure' and that within the latter category three types may be observed:

1. anxious/ambivalent
2. avoidant
3. disorganised/disoriented.

According to Parkes, it is the carrying through of these early patterns of attachment into adult relationships which is a major determinant of grieving patterns later in life. Insecure attachments are a fundamental source of complicated grieving (although not the only source, as Parkes acknowledges) and the focus for therapeutic intervention. This theory explains, for example, why the relationship that was fraught with ambivalence, even hostility, may be more problematic to grieve than one that was generally harmonious. The secure attachment seems to lead to a less complicated grief, although the sadness and loss may be overwhelming for a time.

The consequence of forming attachments, particularly those involving emotional commitment, is the likelihood of experiencing the pain of loss at some point. The notion that reaching the point of being able to 'let go' of the person who has died is a turning point in the grief process, and refusing to let go is a sign that the person is 'stuck' in their grief, was central to grief theory and readily applied by grief counsellors for a long time. Its validity lies at the heart of one of the most vigorously debated theoretical developments in recent work – the theory of continuing bonds. We shall consider the way in which holding on or relinquishing bonds are treated in the theoretical approaches which follow. However, it is important to note that attachment theory brings together facets of two of the earliest approaches to understanding grief – biological explanations and psychoanalytic theory. Elements of both of these have continuing currency in contemporary discussions. The original formulations of each are detailed and theoretically sophisticated and there is no attempt here to do more than highlight a central idea which has been carried forward into current discussions.

Biological explanations

This approach conceptualises grief as a stressor threatening the healthy balance of the organism. The original thinking was set out by Lindemann (1944) and Engel (1961). Between them they described grief as a psychological sickness manifested in a range of physiological symptoms, such as anxiety, and including actual physical illness. These responses are again described by Worden (2003) as the 'affects of grief', and they have been commonly used by grief trainers in helping bereavement counsellors to recognise the 'symptoms' of grief. These early biological explanations categorised responses as 'normal' or 'abnormal' (Engel used the term 'morbid grief') and led to the prevalence of the concept of 'pathological grief'. It is only in the last decade that the term 'pathological' has been replaced by 'complicated' grief, as the diversity of experiences and responses to bereavement have begun to be recognised. Biological explanations also link with 'classical crisis theory' (Caplan, 1961) which, as Thompson has pointed out, has been somewhat neglected in more recent work on grief (N. Thompson, 2002). Classical crisis theory suggests that any threat, loss or challenge to familiar patterns and functioning may cause an upset in the 'organism's' steady state ('homeostasis') to which there is a strong drive to return. The disequilibrium in the meantime is experienced as acute crisis. The idea that there are crisis periods within dying and grief – such as at the time of diagnosis, sometimes the actual point of death, sometimes the point when the implications of bereavement really hit home – is recognised by practitioners, but there has been little theoretical attention to this concept which might assist those offering support to people who are dying and bereaved.

Psychoanalytic approaches

These explanations are rooted in the work of Freud. Freud explained 'melancholia', the sadness and depression of grief, as the work of mourning for the loss of a love object (Freud, 1917). Through mourning, the individual reviews her/his memories of the love object and gradually relinquishes the attachment – that is, the hopes, emotional energy and parts of the self which were invested in the lost relationship. This is not quite the same thing as severing all connections (Small, 2001), although it has been so construed by critics of Freud's theory. Nor does it preclude the notion of retaining the lost object in a reconstituted version of the self, which the following first-hand accounts, provided several decades apart, convey:

> 'The person I am now, in part, is *daughter*. I feel that quite strongly actually.' (Lloyd, 1996, p 305)
>
> 'I still have him somewhere, and though it hurts, it hurts like the sun hurts your eyes … he is with me in a real way.' (Gabrielle Maughan, 1988)
>
> '… she seems to meet me everywhere … I don't mean anything remotely like an apparition or a voice … Rather, a sort of unobtrusive but massive sense that she is, just as much as ever, a fact to be taken into account.' (Lewis, 1966, p 42)

Freud has largely gone out of fashion, particularly among professions such as social work which in the 1970s reacted strongly to the pathologising of individuals and 'medical model' of treatment which had grown out of the application of Freudian theory. Not only, however, is social work beginning to rediscover the significance of health and illness in its social explanations and interventions but grief theory has also begun to highlight again the deep, continuing pain of loss of a loved one which Freud's 'melancholia' captured so acutely.

Stage theories

A number of writers have developed frameworks for understanding grief which describe a linear process, the idea being that, as a general drift, individuals move from the initial impact of the loss to a state where they have assimilated this loss (Averill, 1968; Bowlby, 1980; Rando, 1986; Parkes, 1996; Worden, 2003). These various models actually contain within them two slightly different slants. Worden and Rando identify a number of psychological 'tasks' which the grieving person must undertake in order to move on, where the other theories focus on describing different phases in the process of grief. However, they all have in common the notion of linear progression although both Parkes and Rando emphasise that individuals may go in and out of phases. There are marked similarities between them (and also, with Kubler-Ross's stages of dying). Table 4.1 summarises these models. This notion of grief proceeding via linear stages established itself throughout the

Table 4.1: Stage theories

Kubler-Ross (stages of dying)	*Bowlby (process of mourning)*	*Averill (stages of grief)*	*Parkes (phases of grief)*	*Worden (tasks of mourning)*	*Rando (treatment processes)*
Denial	Numbness	Shock	Numbness	To accept the reality of the loss	Recognise the loss
Anger	Yearning, searching and anger	Despair	Pining	To work through to the pain of grief (2nd edn version)	React to the separation
Bargaining					Recollect and re-experience the deceased and the old assumptive world
Depression	Disorganisation and despair		Depression	To adjust to an environment in which the deceased is missing	Relinquish the old attachments to the deceased and the old assumptive world
Acceptance	Reorganisation	Recovery	Recovery	To emotionally relocate the deceased and move on with life (2nd edn version)	Readjust and move adaptively into the new world without forgetting the old
					Reinvest

1970s and 1980s as the unchallenged wisdom, heavily drawn upon by professionals and trained volunteers alike working with dying and bereaved people.

Rather than describing each model, the following section briefly summarises the key common features within phases and the juxtaposition of tasks. The process usually begins with the immediate impact of the death. However, work on anticipatory mourning suggests that it may be earlier, for example on being told the terminal diagnosis or at the point when the 'essence' of the person appears to have diminished through physical and intellectual deterioration such that the relationship as it was has ceased. Numbness and shock are said to predominate and the full force of feelings not felt, or not felt continuously. As the person grapples with the reality of the death, however (and this may in part be through the social rituals discussed earlier and events such as the funeral), he or she begins to recognise the loss that they have incurred. There is a strong drive to deny this reality. This might be a denial that the person has actually died (and this can be made particularly difficult to accept when there is uncertainty surrounding the announcement, as in deaths in overseas conflict zones, or where the bereaved is physically distanced from, or excluded from, the events immediately before and after the death). Or the denial might manifest itself as a refusal to believe that the situation is irreversible. Or the bereaved person may deny to themselves the significance of the death for their future life.

This young mother, speaking about the death of her husband three years earlier, expresses very well how denial and realisation go hand in hand:

> '… then there was the realisation one day, although I had accepted that he'd died, that he really, really wasn't coming back, and it didn't matter how much I talked about it and how much I wished and wanted, he wasn't going to come back.' (Young widow, author's previously unreported data)

As reality begins to bite, however, the bereaved person begins to experience the intense pain of loss, to pine or yearn for what has been lost (both the person and their 'old world') and to try to assuage these feelings by seeking out the person who has gone. Some people describe aimless wandering, others finding themselves in places where they might normally have expected to be with their deceased partner, and Parkes likens this 'searching behaviour' to the frantic searching, alternating with lifeless behaviour, which can be observed in some animals that have lost their mate. For others, their pining may be reflected in maintaining the 'presence' of the person who has gone, either through routines (such as setting their place at the table), leaving some graphic reminder (such as an answerphone message or half-finished task) or continuing to include them in conversation as though they were still alive. Every disappointed 'search' or jolt of realisation, serves to confirm that the person and the old life have gone, and a new existence must replace it.

The process of grappling with this new life is sometimes seen as the real 'work' of grief, characterised by both disorganisation, as the bereaved person struggles to adjust and make changes necessary to survive without the person who has died, but also periods of depression and sometimes despair that they cannot, or do not wish to, go on. Often the bereaved person becomes immersed in reviewing their former life and relationship and this may involve further recognition of what exactly has been lost, such that the raw pain of grief surfaces. The task of readjustment may be made more difficult by those around, who are keen to see the bereaved person establish a new life but find it difficult to watch, or may actively disapprove of, them spending time on recollection and review, particularly when this stirs up painful feelings. By contrast, in some non-western cultures, the activity of shared recollection, when family and friends get together, is customary. The degree of disruption and disorganisation experienced varies according to, among other things, the extent to which the bereaved person had shared their 'life space' and identity with the person who has died. For example, it is likely to be greater for the mother of a very young baby, or for the surviving spouse in a couple who also worked together and shared the same social circle, such that their lives overlapped completely.

As the bereaved person begins to establish their new life without the person who has died, their focus begins to change. Emotional and psychological energy, which they had been pouring into recollecting and grieving what has been lost, is channelled into the present and eventually into making plans for the future. This renewed interest in life accompanied by reorganised behaviour, is described as recovery and reinvestment. Crucially, it involves relinquishing the old attachments. This has often been translated, particularly in reductionist paraphrasing, into 'letting go' – the bone of contention with proponents of 'continuing bonds' theory (see later discussion). However, a point which critics of the idea of 'relinquishing bonds' often ignore is that a more careful reading of these stage theorists reveals that they are talking more about reworking these attachments into their new world, than cutting the ties completely. Parkes talks about recovery involving resurrection and rediscovery of the relationship, sometimes through a concrete means such as completing a project which had been important to the lost person or undertaking alone something which had been a joint aspiration, and sometimes through incorporation of the shared life into the new identity. This concept of 'resurrection', as the bereaved person's experience of the ongoing contribution of the person who has died, is also described by Lindemann (1976).

Rehearsing this summary account and seeing the various stage theories set out in tabular fashion (Table 4.1) makes immediately obvious what the problem is with this form of theoretical modelling. The complex phenomenon of grief does not fit neatly into boxes and there is a great danger of misunderstanding the individual experience when any one of these models is applied as a template. This does not mean that they do not have value, and they have, in fact, contributed a great deal to our understanding of grief. As Small points out, descriptive accounts derived from a mixture of clinical practice and empirical research (but more particularly the former) were never meant to be applied prescriptively (Small, 2001). However, substantial criticisms have been made of stage theories on two counts: (i) because they are culturally monolithic, and (ii) because the counterpoint of describing a 'normal' progression through grief is that some people are deemed to get 'stuck' in a particular phase (for example, never really accepting that the person has gone) or to actively resist a particular task (for example, resisting learning new skills required to adapt to their new environment). While both issues may apply and be the source of complicated grieving, the criticism is that the distinction made between 'normal' and 'abnormal' grief is too clear-cut and the notion of 'progression' applied too rigidly. Possibly the biggest challenge to this has come from work with bereaved parents, where chronic grief as 'normal' is repeatedly reported.

Psychosocial transition

Before we move away from the work of Colin Murray Parkes, I want to highlight his work on bereavement as psychosocial transition (Parkes, 1993). Not only does this work seem to me to be theoretically compelling, it also offers a very useful framework for the practitioner. This is based on the idea that the individual experiences and makes sense of their world through a series of 'assumptive models'. These are constructed for both their *internal* world – the person's inner reality, used to manage intra-psychic processes – and their *external* world – the reality of the outside world, used to manage their relations with the outside. Bereavement represents a threat to both sets of models, and Parkes suggests that it is the interaction between the individual's inner and outer worlds that shapes their bereavement experience. The process of relinquishing or adjusting old models and establishing new ones to make sense of the altered reality (inner and outer) is described by Parkes as 'psychosocial transition'. It is through grieving that the person reviews and adjusts or replaces their inner models, and it is through social interaction and finding their new social identity, sometimes aided by the formal social rituals surrounding death, that they develop new assumptive models to negotiate the outside world.

There is for me one striking omission from the theory of bereavement as psychosocial transition, although it is a dimension which can be inferred from the way in which Parkes explains it. The bereaved person has also to find new ways of understanding their sense of 'being': in other words bereavement also threatens their *existential* models. This may result in a strengthening of existing models, rediscovery of those formerly held, or discarding existing models and seeking to establish new ones (Lloyd, 1996). From my work on spiritual issues in dying and bereavement I would suggest three adaptations of Parkes' model:

- It should be extended to encompass psychosocial-existential transition.
- It should parallel in the psychological and social realms the notion of an existential search, with the possibility that the resulting adjustments may involve strengthening existing models or returning to former models as well as establishing new ones.

- It should be applied to the process of dying, which (in my view) is currently under-theorised.

Dual process

A break with this tradition of a linear process of grief occurred with the theory of 'dual process' put forward by Stroebe and Schut (1999). They argue that there are two axes simultaneously present in people's response to bereavement – *loss orientation* and *restoration orientation* – and bereaved people oscillate between them. Stroebe arrived at this theory through puzzling over the problem of the difference between reviewing the lost relationship, a common activity in grief, and obsessive grief, which is generally recognised as unhelpful. The development of dual process, sometimes described as 'two track' models (Malkinson et al, 2006), also continues to be informed by work which suggests that recovery may be inhibited by the expression of negative emotion and is hastened by positive emotions and thinking associated with ongoing functioning (Bonanno, 2001). Dual process theory suggests that the grieving person will focus on 'restoration' plans and activities when focusing on the loss becomes too much to bear. Individuals will have their own unique balance between loss and restoration, although orienting towards one at the expense of the other is seen to be an indication of either chronic grief (overly loss-oriented) or inhibited grief (overly restoration-oriented). There are some suggestions that gender and cultural influences may incline the individual more towards one form of coping than the other, but this evidence is as yet hesitant. The following quote from a male school teacher, talking about his return to work after his baby daughter's death, indicates how complex is the question of gender 'styles' and their interaction with grief in western culture:

> 'I think I'm perhaps just typical male in the sense that I don't think I open myself up very much to telling people how I felt. I had great difficulties with my male colleagues at work, it was mainly females who would keep asking me how [wife] was and asking me questions which enabled me to open up a little bit, and I remember vividly being in a situation with six or seven males around a table … and I mentioned one of the problems has been that a lot of people I know obviously feel great sadness etc. but can't bring themselves to speak about it in case they upset me. I remember virtually to a man every single one of them had a great surge of relief, "Oh yes, yes …" and then the lid was on again.' (Author's previously unpublished data)

Although dual process is not a linear model, its creators acknowledge that the tendency to focus on loss will be stronger in the early days of bereavement, with the balance shifting towards restoration as time goes on. This is perhaps not a long way off the accounts from stage theory which allow for people going in and out of phases. Reports of therapeutic interventions using the dual process model are still relatively rare. One study from Israel found it necessary to focus on the loss, even where there was initial resistance, in order to make progress on the restoration of functioning (Malkinson et al, 2006). The reason for this was because a reworked ongoing relationship with the person who had died was central to restoring general functioning. It is to the question of maintaining, rather than relinquishing, attachments to which we now turn, since the theory of 'continuing bonds' has assumed important status in the current discourse on grief.

Continuing bonds

In the 1990s evidence began to emerge that for many bereaved people, maintaining connections with the person who had died was a core aspect of their ongoing functioning and contributed to their adjustment. The theory of 'continuing bonds', as it has come to be called, is particularly associated with the work of Dennis Klass, an American bereavement researcher and psychotherapist (Klass et al, 1996). There is already evidence that continuing bonds is being adopted by some, particularly in the caring professions, as the new orthodoxy replacing the long-held accepted wisdom of stage theory and 'letting go'. Klass himself has pointed out that (as with the stage theory) 'continuing bonds' was never meant to be applied prescriptively – as a formula for healthy grieving – but was simply a description of what he and other researchers had observed (Klass, 2006). Klass had originally undertaken an ethnographic study of support groups for bereaved parents (Klass, 1988), and his evidence concurs with that collected anecdotally by workers facilitating such groups, which continuously suggested that grieving over a child commonly shows no signs of abating at the first-year anniversary (normally seen as something of a milestone in stage theory) and that the notion of 'letting go' is something that bereaved parents just cannot contemplate (Osterweis et al, 1984).

In fact it is the nature of attachments and bonds and the ways in which relinquishing or retaining them promotes or hinders healthy adjustment that have always been the core of bereavement research (Stroebe and Schut, 2005; Field, 2006). These issues continue to be at the heart of the current debate surrounding continuing bonds. The crucial question is whether or not retaining attachments is an adaptive or maladaptive response to bereavement, since obsessive clinging to memories and maintaining tangible reminders in a 'frozen' state (for example the room in which nothing must be touched but is kept almost as a 'shrine') represents, according to attachment theorists, one of the forms of complicated grief. Some researchers do not see 'continuing bonds' as a challenge to attachment theories of grief, arguing that attachment theory provides a framework which accommodates the functionality of continuing bonds by categorising different forms of attachment and their implications for loss (Field et al, 2005). Stroebe and Schut argue that continuing bonds theorists may have demonstrated that retaining attachments is part of normal grief, but they have not demonstrated that such behaviour *promotes* healthy grieving (Stroebe and Schut, 2005).

Klass counters that this was never the argument; it happens and it may or may not be helpful, in the same way as any attachment may be the source of well-being or the root of emotional and mental health problems: 'the criteria for the health of an interpersonal bond are the same whether the bond is between living people or between living people and dead people' (Klass, 2006, p. 845).

Boerner and Heckhausen (2003) drawing on work from others, suggest that for continuing bonds to assist with grief, the former attachments must be 'transformed' rather than retained.

The crucial issue, for Klass, is that we have moved on from assuming that maintaining bonds is per se unhealthy. Attachment theorists are rather more concerned to establish a 'normative course' for continuing bonds, implying that the phenomenon of individuals who cling unhealthily to attachments, or whose grief process is complicated by previous unhealthy attachments, remains the greater problem (Field et al, 2005). Reisman concludes that retaining connections with 'higher order postulates' – that is, fundamental assumptions concerned with more abstract frameworks – is adaptive, whereas clinging to 'lower order postulates' – that is, more concrete frameworks belonging to a particular situation or set of circumstances – is maladaptive. The latter are normally a tailored response and have to adjust to the new situation occasioned by the bereavement (Reisman, 2001). On the basis of my own work discussed earlier, I would suggest that 'higher order postulates' also have to be reworked. My research also found that people who could find no meaningful connections with more abstract frameworks struggled more than most: 'I'm not religious, but don't get me wrong, I pray every night ... I'm confused, very confused ... I'm willing to try anything, I am' (Lloyd, 1996, p 307).

Complicated grief

A substantial section of current bereavement research is concerned with grief that is particularly complicated. Thus far we have been considering theories about the ways in which people deal with grief, which have in common the notion that while grief is a 'normal' human reaction, it is always difficult and the potential for it to be particularly problematic is high. At one time the distinction was made between 'normal' and 'pathological' grief. However, criticism of overly prescriptive models of grieving and suggestions that a diversity of response is ordinarily present, as well as the impact of considerable cultural differences, has led to the term 'complicated grieving' replacing the notion of 'pathological' grief. Most importantly, there is acknowledgment that no clear-cut division exists between the categories of 'normal' and 'complicated', although complicated grief continues to be linked to a psychiatric perspective (Neimeyer et al, 2002).[2] Between 10 and 20 per cent of bereaved people are thought to experience significant difficulty in dealing with their loss (Prigerson and Jacobs, 2001) and a stream of ongoing work is concerned with refining previous understandings of what was variously termed 'morbid', 'abnormal' or 'pathological' (Jacobs et al, 2000). This can be organised into three broad categories which define or give rise to complicated grief: *affectual*, *attachment-related* and *situational*. Spanning both the attachment-related and situational categories of complicated grief, is a category defined by some theorists as *traumatic grief*, which proponents are at pains to point out is distinct from post-traumatic stress disorder but sufficiently problematic to warrant the drawing up of specific diagnostic criteria. Two pathways are said to lead to traumatic grief: bereavement resulting from sudden, violent or horrific death; and bereavement experienced by individuals whose attachment styles leave them particularly vulnerable to separation and loss (Jacobs et al, 2000).

Problems related to the affects of grief

Throughout the history of bereavement research, one of its features has been to describe grief in all its manifestations. This can be particularly useful for practitioners in raising their awareness of the range of feelings and behaviours that might normally be experienced in grief, where, without personal experience to help them understand, they might otherwise have thought it indicative of malfunctioning or problematic behaviour. Much misunderstanding and inaccurate assessment occurs because the impact of grief on a service user's behaviour is not acknowledged (Lloyd, 1992). Maureen Oswin's study of bereavement among learning-disabled people (Oswin, 1991) provides many examples of this: outbursts of anger on being admitted to residential care following the death of a parent earns the learning-disabled person the label of 'challenging behaviour', for example. It can also be useful to be able to reassure the bereaved person that they are not going mad – although they may, as Shakespeare terms it, be 'maddened' by grief.

Worden divides these indicators of grief into *feelings*, *physical sensations*, *cognitions* and *behaviours* (Table 4.2). Again, the cautionary note must be sounded: it should

Table 4.2: Worden's affects of grief

Feelings
- Sadness
- Anger
- Guilt/self-reproach
- Anxiety
- Loneliness
- Helplessness
- Emancipation
- Relief
- Numbness

Physical sensations
- Hollowness in stomach
- Tightness in chest
- Tightness in throat
- Oversensitivity to noise
- Sense of depersonalisation
- Breathlessness
- Weakness
- Lack of energy
- Dry mouth

Cognitions
- Disbelief
- Confusion
- Preoccupation
- Sense of deceased's presence
- Hallucinations

Behaviours
- Sleep disturbances
- Appetite disturbances
- Absent-minded behaviour
- Social withdrawal
- Dreams of deceased
- Avoiding reminders
- Searching and calling out for deceased
- Sighing
- Restless overactivity
- Crying
- Visiting reminders/carrying reminder objects
- Treasuring objects

not be assumed that the bereaved person *must* experience everything on the list, simply that they *might*. Equally, it should not be assumed that a particular physical disturbance is caused by grief; it might need (or benefit from) medical attention but, equally, it might turn out to be psychosomatic in origin.

The picture of the affects of 'normal' grief is used as one means of indicating complicated grief. This category of complicated grief is where symptom distress is excessive, prolonged and seriously functionally debilitating. So, for example, anger, guilt, avoiding reminders or, conversely, desperately maintaining them, or disbelief, are features which seem particularly prone to be carried to excess and to remain at the initial levels of high emotional disturbance. This can be the clue to the source of the complication. The following case illustrates this well.

Mandy was a 30-year-old woman with a learning disability who had entered residential care on the death of her mother. After a period of some disruption, involving a number of moves, she settled in a supported flat in the community. She appeared to be managing OK except for the fact that she carried round with her a set of photographs from her previous life and became hysterical if separated from them, even for a moment. She was assigned a key worker who talked with her about the photographs and the memories they evoked, and visited with her significant places depicted in them. Eventually Mandy put the photographs away in a drawer, although they were always brought out to show to a new visitor.

Problematic attachments

Attachment theorists start from the premise that insecure attachments predispose the individual to a complicated bereavement reaction. They are then concerned with two aspects of complicated grief: the relationship between particular types of insecure attachments and the loss experience, and the specific areas for therapeutic intervention which this indicates. Linking this to his three categories of insecure attachments (see p 67 above). Parkes (2006) suggests key therapeutic tasks arising from the nature of these attachments.

- Avoidant 'types' may need permission to grieve and continuing reassurance as they embark on what is for them a risky process.
- Anxious/ambivalent 'types' may need permission to stop active grieving and reassurance that they are not betraying their love for the person who has died in so doing.
- Disorganised 'types' may need both permission to grieve and to draw a line under some aspects; they are likely to need considerable reassurance because the process in itself may feel chaotic.

Situations which create complications

Some bereavements incorporate a range of social, psychological and emotional features, which predispose the individual to complicated grief. Some also present a particular existential challenge.

One feature of the situational category of complicated grief is that the loss experienced by the bereaved person is not recognised by those around them; this may include the immediate family as well as the wider community. Ken Doka has referred to this as *disenfranchised grief* (Doka, 2001). Thus the bereaved person has no social sanction for their grief. Doka suggests that it may be the griever, the relationship or the loss which is disenfranchised. Either the bereaved person is not assumed to experience grief (as is often the case for people with a learning disability or dementia), or the relationship is one which is secret (as in an extra-marital affair) or stigmatised (commonly the experience in the past for people in same-sex relationships, who may still be pushed to one side by the family of their partner). Or the loss is not recognised as a bereavement (as in a miscarriage – and also for the 'father', when his partner miscarries). In such circumstances, the griever is robbed of a social context for their grief, as well as the social status of bereaved person, making the negotiation of the psychosocial transition particularly difficult. Often they are excluded from the important social rituals surrounding the death. A study in Germany found that disenfranchised grievers were more likely than other bereaved people to keep up old social routines (such as a weekly restaurant meal) thus creating their own rituals (Weiser and Ochsmann, 2005).

What should also be remembered is that the circumstances of 'disenfranchised' grief commonly include ambivalence, ambiguity, guilt, anxiety, insecurity and diminished self-esteem on the part of the bereaved person, either as a pre-existing condition or occasioned by the circumstances of the death. The following case from my own practice as a social worker illustrates this accumulation of factors contributing to complicated grief. The case also demonstrates something that is widely 'known' but little written about (except in relation to bereaved parents). A complicated grief reaction in one family member has significant knock-on effects for others, and also hinders the resolution of coexisting problems. In the following case, unravelling the consequences of sexual abuse within the family was made even more painful and resistant to therapeutic intervention by the mother's complicated grief.

A 15-year-old boy was referred to the hospital social worker because of repeated admissions for urinary problems for which no underlying cause could be found. It transpired that the father was serving a prison sentence for sexually abusing his daughter and son. The mother disclosed to the social worker that she had been engaged in an affair for several years prior to the abuse coming to light. Her lover had died following a heart attack which occurred whilst they were out together, and in her panic about discovery, she had called an ambulance and left him alone. Her grief was complicated not only by the fact that she could not show her feelings to her family (who did not know of the affair) but also by extreme guilt about her behaviour during the affair and at her lover's death.

Overall we can conclude that, although the complicated grief may belong predominantly to one or other of the categories outlined, there are likely to be features of each category involved for any person who requires professional intervention. There is continuing discussion about the most effective forms of intervention, with one body of work suggesting that even complicated and traumatic grief reactions may be best left to informal processes and supports, and we should not underestimate most people's capacity to deal with grief in their own way (Bonanno, 2004). Others suggest that focusing on the negative emotions of grief is not helpful and cognitive behavioural therapies may be more effective (Bonanno et al, 1995; Matthews and Marwitt, 2004). Perhaps counter to the view that most people do not need professional intervention is the experience of non-specialist workers: that people often raise grief-related issues alongside some other problem, implying that they are not able to get the support they need outside of the professional encounter (Lloyd, 1992). In this circumstance, the health and social care worker can be seen to be 'standing in' for the friend or neighbour, thus offering a different form of help to the focused clinical grief intervention. Sometimes, when an unresolved loss from the past is reactivated by a current crisis, it becomes clear that in addressing the two simultaneously, a form of grief therapy is being offered (Lloyd, 1992).

Meaning-making

The theory promoted by Neimeyer (2001), which sees grief as essentially a process of meaning reconstruction, belongs to more recent work. Significant loss represents a major challenge to the personal meanings which the individual has established and these must be renegotiated and reconstructed after bereavement. This has similarities with Marris's classic work on loss and change, in which he makes connections between a sense of meaninglessness and overall disorientation and chaos (Marris, 1974). The applicability of this concept to death has been drawn out elsewhere (Rowe, 1989; Lloyd, 1992). In its juxtaposition of the psychological and social contexts for the creation of the individual's unique 'meaning set' (my term), meaning reconstruction is not unlike the understanding of bereavement as psychosocial transition. However, it belongs to the constructivist school of thought, which sees the individual as an active learner and agent in their own process of change. The different processes of sense-making, benefit-finding and identity reconstruction are separately identified, combined by the bereaved person in what Neimeyer describes as grief self-narratives (Neimeyer and Anderson, 2002). This is the way in which bereaved people organise the account of their loss in the context of their life as a whole, all the while seeking to establish new meanings or accommodations of the old disrupted ones. This woman from my own study articulates her search to recreate the narrative: 'There was a sense of, "This isn't in the script" ... your life's got to find structure and meaning' (Lloyd, 1996, p 301).

Although meaning-making is applicable across the board, it might be seen to have particular relevance for individuals at risk of a complicated grief reaction, since one of the key features has been found to be the inability to make sense of what has happened. Neimeyer and colleagues, in a study of 506 bereaved young adults with personal and circumstantial characteristics which put them at risk, found that active engagement with all three dimensions of meaning reconstruction – sense-making, benefit-finding and identity reconstruction – significantly moderated their distress. They also found that strong continuing bonds served to heighten distress, but only if the individual was unable to make any sense of the loss (Neimeyer et al, 2006).

The existential search

Research into transcendental experiences has found that well over half of the general population in the UK claim to have had such experiences, although not all would term them religious (Hardy, 1979). Illness, the prospect of death and bereavement were significant triggers. A survey of social workers in the US, followed by a replicated study in the UK, found that of the four areas of social work practice in which social workers expressed the greatest approval for raising the topic of spirituality, three were related to loss and death – terminal illness, bereavement and in situations of natural disaster. Religion was seen as slightly less appropriate. This finding is particularly interesting for the UK, because social workers there remain wary of the topics of spirituality and religion (Holloway, 2007), yet these workers are clearly identifying something different about working with people who are dying or bereaved. In a series of interviews exploring the impact of terminal illness or bereavement on their thinking and outlook, 22 of the 23 people I interviewed at least touched on existential issues, and eleven explored in some detail their personal philosophy, spirituality or religious beliefs (Lloyd, 1996).

Meaning reconstruction is clearly at the heart of this process, but we should not assume that meaning-making and the existential search are entirely synonymous, or that everyone engages with a continuing quest about the meaning of their whole existence and the human condition. Lifton (1979) identified five 'modes of death transcendence' – the *bio-social*, *creative*, *religious*, *nature* and the *mystical*. These are spheres of activity and ways of engaging with the problem which the individual uses to 'transcend' the challenge to their modus operandi created by the proximity of death. Only the religious and the mystical may encompass the existential search although all modes may be used in the reconstruction of meaning. Lifton described the 'religious mode' as identifying and deriving support from a particular religious explanation. Over half of my respondents were able to draw support from previously held or handed-down childhood religious beliefs, but the following quotations illustrate that this did not involve any prolonged or probing search:

> 'When you've been brought up with it you don't have to reach out.'
>
> 'Now whether you like to think that you're going to see them again one day, I don't know. I don't care anyway, that's what I want to think and that's what I believe.' (Lloyd, 1996, p 300)

Lifton's 'mystical mode' involves a shift from cognitive to experiential perception. Six of my respondents explored their search for meaning which involved formulating or reformulating their 'belief' structures in the teeth of experience. Two others indicated that they had gone through this process on more than one occasion previously when faced with loss, and had now arrived at a position where their framework of belief could encompass the present experience. Two others indicated that they felt hopelessly adrift in a sea of chaos and meaninglessness.

It is important to understand how these positions might relate to the overall experience of grief and the contribution which existential issues might make to complicated grieving. The last two women were each receiving grief therapy but made faltering connections between their inability to make progress with their emotional problems and the failure of the counselling sessions to address their existential despair:

> 'I've no faith in life to be quite honest … without faith you can't go very far.' (Lloyd, 1996, p 306)
>
> 'I'm confused, very confused.' (Lloyd, 1996, p 307)

Themes of punishment (which were also strong in these women's narratives), with a resulting loss of trust and profound sense of alienation, have been noted as a feature of complicated grief resulting from traumatic loss (McBride and Armstrong, 1995).

We discussed earlier in this chapter how crisis may form part of the dying or bereaved person's experience. Loss of religious faith has been noted as a common response to terminal illness and bereavement, as much as for some people beliefs are strengthened (Lloyd, 1996; Gibson, 2006). What is less considered is the existential search instigated when previously held beliefs prove unsatisfactory in the crisis, but the individual needs to find a new framework of 'belief' within which to locate their experience. Four women in my study indicated the existential nature of their crisis, describing this search for meaning and 'answers' as central to their distress as well as to their ability to integrate the loss and emerge from the crisis. They displayed a complex interpretation of both question and answer, looking to professional helpers for guidance in searching for their own meanings rather than 'answers'. Only one was in ongoing contact with a religious professional, whom she had sought out specifically because she had not found the help she needed elsewhere and thought that he, if anyone, should be used to this sort of process.

In general, it can be noted that existential issues are stronger where the death is untimely or appears particularly 'unfair'. It is common, for example, for grandparents to express a sense that they should not still be here, that they wish it had been them, when their adult child has died leaving a young family. In my survey of hospital social workers and chaplains, the social workers working with child death all identified existential concerns as one of the three distinguishing features of their work. In the next section, we see that they feature strongly in deaths whose individual and social circumstances make them particularly difficult to grieve.

Special deaths

There are some categories of death which are commonly recognised as being particularly difficult for the bereaved to cope with. This is because the deaths themselves combine circumstances and features which significantly complicate the grief reaction, irrespective of the individual features of the bereaved person or their relationship with the person who has died. Complications such as insecure attachments may well be added into the equation. For these reasons, these deaths are sometimes termed 'special'.[3] Special deaths are defined as those which incur a high level of psychosocial trauma; they may be socially stigmatising or existentially problematic, and frequently both; the grief is often 'disenfranchised' (see earlier discussion).

Table 4.3: Special deaths

Feature	Example
Psychosocial trauma	Murder
Social stigma	Drug overdose
Existential problems	Child death
Disenfranchised grief	Secret relationship

Recognised special deaths

For some time now, it has been recognised that there are three groups whose especial needs are highly likely to require professional help: bereaved parents, persons bereaved through suicide, and the bereaved child. Considerable attention has been paid to developing the skills and interventive methods designed to assist them in their grief. This has resulted in a degree of public awareness of the problems for bereaved people in these categories, which may at least reduce the likelihood of their pain being made worse by insensitive comments and behaviour of those around them. Nevertheless, these bereavements remain amongst the hardest to deal with, and chronic and complicated grief are common. Moreover, we are increasingly seeing parental bereavement occurring in the contexts of one or other of the special deaths discussed here. For example, there is a growth in teenage suicide; there have been a number of cases in the past decade of shootings in schools; drug-users are, in the majority, relatively young and the younger people are more likely to die from an accidental overdose or unexpected reaction while experimenting; and, although still mercifully rare, there is an increase in child abductions resulting in death.

The bereaved parent

Death of a child, first and foremost for the parents, is an overturning of the expected order of events, destroying not only their present, but their hopes and expectations for the future. Existential issues are common. Not only is the death of a child untimely, it also represents loss of part of oneself and one's partner. Chronic and complicated grief is common, and it is now recognised that 'resolution' is a meaningless goal; learning to live with the loss and accommodate its ongoing implications is as much as most bereaved parents aim for. The stage of attachment at which the child dies is significant in shaping the experience of grief; for example, the death of a teenager or toddler, stages in the parent–child relationship commonly marked by conflict, may leave the parent particularly open to regret. The way in which the child dies may also significantly shape the bereavement experience. Children and young people die through accident, acute illness or as a result of a life-threatening condition, often congenital. There may be guilt or recriminations against the partner, and relationship breakdown is high after the death of a child. Where parents have been intensively involved in the care of a sick child, exhaustion, distress at watching but being unable to prevent the child's suffering, and problems arising in the family through perceived neglect of other children, are common in the ensuing bereavement period. The impact on family dynamics, with patterns such as idealising the dead child; turning surviving children into replacements who must assume the dead sibling's characteristics; and sometimes having another baby who literally becomes the replacement, with consequences for their development in their own right, pose further risks to the family. A systems theory approach to understanding the needs of families experiencing bereavement works from the perspective that the family as an organism is hurt and needs to find a new equilibrium.

Suicide

The overwhelming problem for the person bereaved through suicide is the sense of rejection, that they, and their relationship, were not enough for the person to want to live. Moreover, suicide is in some sense felt as a rejection of the wider community and society, thus compounding the inhibition that others might feel in offering support to the most immediately bereaved. People bereaved through suicide appear to experience the range of grief reactions but often in exaggerated form, combined with particular features. A sense of abandonment and rejection may result in very low self-esteem; this can be particularly damaging for a child whose parent commits suicide. Guilt arising from the belief that they played some part in the person's decision to commit suicide, or that they should have prevented it, may lead to self-punishing behaviour. Often there will be denial that the death was a result of suicide, made all the more likely in circumstances where there is some doubt, but often leading to distorted communications within the surviving family. The strong stigma surrounding suicide may cause the person to feel there is no one to whom they can talk about what happened, their feelings around the death and the loss.

The bereaved child

The developmental stage of the child when the death of a significant person occurs is possibly the most significant factor determining how grief is experienced and expressed. For infants and very young children, the crucial factor in their adjustment appears to be the quality of substitute care if a parent or other carer dies, and the degree to which the child's routine is disturbed. For the older child, the major complication is that adults frequently try to protect the child from the truth, and the child may be excluded from significant events like the funeral. Where the child is old enough to understand causality he or she may feel guilty that some aspect of their behaviour, or a particular incident, contributed to, or brought about, the illness and/or death. It is suggested that the child's concept of death develops in stages and this also affects the way in which they understand the loss and are able to grieve. For example, very young children do not understand death to be irreversible, a perception which may well be reinforced by the 'fantasy dying' played out in TV and film dramas. A later stage is the personification of death, in which the reality of death is understood but is something to be deeply feared, as a threatening presence. Such fears may well relate to night terrors with the child refusing to go to bed or sleep in their own room after a bereavement. Stories in the media of child abductions are likely to confirm such fears. As the child begins to reach a mature concept of death, he or she comes also to understand that death is universal and irreversible.

Loss of a significant person through death in childhood has been correlated with mental health problems in adulthood, when combined with other risk factors. However, with the right support children can survive the death of a parent, and mourning, if begun at the time, may be completed later in life, usually around a significant event or period in the young person's or adult's life, such as graduating from college. Common complications are that the child may over-identify with the parent who has died and this may hinder their personal development. Some children may fear that they will not survive beyond the age at which the parent died or even be driven to repeat a behaviour such as suicide. Death of a sibling is complicated by the existence of sibling rivalry and by parents seeking to replace the dead child by bestowing their characteristics on a surviving child.

The most important point in assisting a child with grief is that their mourning should be recognised, that adults around the child should also understand that it may take place over a different timescale from their own and that the manifestations of grief will be different – for example, the child going out to play with friends straight after the funeral does not mean that they are unaffected. Bowlby (1980) identifies three favourable conditions to facilitate a child's grief:

- The child is given accurate information and the opportunity to enquire later.
- There is open communication within the family and the surviving parent(s) is sensitive to the child's needs.
- A pattern of healthy family relationships existed prior to the death.

However, it is important that this openness meets the child's needs. Aitkenhead (2005) provides a moving account of the death of her mother, whom she only began to grieve for as an adult. Although her mother's cancer was openly discussed in the family, sorrow and grief went against the positive approach which her parents were determined to pursue and were not allowed (Aitkenhead, 2005). Thus, a crucial part of assisting the child to grieve lies in supporting the parents, so that they are able to see and respond to the child's needs, at the same time as they are themselves grieving. A wider social network to support the family, including other adults in the family who are close to the child, can be immensely helpful. Professional involvement giving the child space away from the family and encouraging them to express their feelings through play therapy and other direct therapeutic techniques may also be employed. Such approaches may be the only possibilities open to children suffering traumatic losses such as those orphaned in war, disaster and the AIDS pandemic, of whose needs we are becoming increasingly aware. For these children, a supportive community substituting for the family is essential in which to nurture their slow recovery.

Special deaths in late modernity

The late twentieth and early twenty-first centuries have seen an escalation in deaths which combine a number of the features of special deaths, and, in addition, are complicated by the sociopolitical context of contemporary society (Guy and Holloway, 2007). These deaths tend to be in the public eye, the private agony being played out in the media, only to be forgotten once the story has peaked, leaving the close bereaved to struggle on alone. In mass deaths, or where particular local communities are affected, there may be continuing support and solidarity from those sharing the impact and grief, but the sense of isolation for these 'grieving communities' from the rest of the world may be just as profound. These special deaths of late modernity are distinguished by being caught up in those features of contemporary death which we discussed in Chapter One. These crucially determine the grief experience of those most closely affected. These distinguishing characteristics can be summarised as follows:

- The social context is problematic and is also of public concern.

- There is media interest, either in the actual death, or in the social or political problem which lies behind it, or sometimes in both aspects.
- There is dissonance between the public representation and private story.
- They represent a threat to the ontological security of the individual and society.
- The bereaved have a strong need to find moral purpose and meaning arising from the event.
- These deaths are outside of the mainstream.

Table 4.4: Special deaths of late modernity

Feature	Example
Public issue	Man-made disaster
Media interest	Serial killings
Public–private clash	Death occasioned by lifestyle of which family unaware
Threaten ontological security	Terrorist incident
Search for moral purpose	Sectarian killing
Alien/marginalised	Drug overdose

Although the examples in Table 4.4 suggest examples of deaths where one particular feature is central, the key point about these deaths is that they each share elements of the whole phenomenon. There is a small, but growing, literature on bereavement through drug-related deaths, mass disaster, murder, terrorist attacks and hostage-taking. Understanding of the needs of gay and lesbian partners where the partner has died of AIDS is a little more established, but the impact of the AIDS pandemic experienced in parts of Africa has been little researched from the point of view of the scale of loss. Unlike much of the 'opening up of death' through media coverage of the topic, these deaths are not ones with which most people connect, although they may be both horrified and fascinated by them. At the same time, these 'special' deaths are an increasing part of the cumulative experience of contemporary death and may be a significant element of the recent history of migrants from war zones, whose presence is a feature of contemporary pluralist societies.

Grief across cultures

The theories discussed in this chapter have without exception originated in western thought and been influenced by the context of family life in western societies. Only one – the theory of continuing bonds – has made explicit theoretical connection, as it developed, to eastern thinking and traditions (Klass and Goss, 1999). Despite taking the social context of modern death as its starting point, bereavement theory has then largely focused on the individual psychological state. We are only gradually acknowledging that these models of individual bereavement might not have universal currency in different social contexts and that this is particularly important for health and social care professionals who find themselves working with someone from another culture or caught between cultures, as is often the case for second and subsequent generations in immigrant communities.

Much of the attempt to understand grief across cultures consists of descriptive accounts of different rituals and practices, and the belief systems within which they are located (Irish, 1993; Parkes et al, 1996). Important as these are, they tell us little about the subjective grief experience of the individual within that culture, which is particularly important for those people who find themselves operating in a cross-cultural context. Rosenblatt suggests that the individual would not engage in culturally prescribed behaviours if they did not assist in expressing their grief and therefore we may assume that particular rituals reflect the ways of understanding and dealing with grief in a particular society that are appropriate for its members (Rosenblatt, 1993). However, Gunaratnam (1997) suggests that confusing public behaviours with private grief results in assumptions being made about the individual's grief and the social support available to them, which may not accord with their needs. A rare example of an attempt to uncover the individual grief experience is provided by Eisenbruch, who investigated variations in the ascription of meaning within different cultural contexts (Eisenbruch, 1984a and 1984b).

However, this may be the wrong track to follow. While some commentators argue that there are greater similarities than differences in the bereavement experience across cultures (Deeken, 2004) and in the approaches to death and dying (Holloway, 2006a), a core difference in the starting points of eastern and western philosophy can be noted. Whereas the west is oriented towards individualism and autonomy, the starting point in many Asian and eastern cultures is communitarian values and social and familial duty (one of the notable things about the Asian tsunami was the way westerners were struck by the concern shown for themselves by the local people despite having suffered immense losses themselves). These influences can be seen in the attitudes to death and social expectations surrounding bereavement in each type of society (Hsu et al, 2004; Payne et al, 2005). However, in a world in which cultural diversity within societies is increasingly the norm, and individuals experiencing social transitions or straddling cultures is a common feature, it is essential that we seek to understand the way in which individual and social perspectives are integrated.

The body of material exploring bereavement across cultures is still remarkably thin. Nevertheless, it is possible to pull out some broad points to further our understanding.

First, the ontological assumptions underpinning culturally prescribed patterns of dying and mourning are of crucial importance. Although secularism can be recognised as a global trend, its coexistence with traditional beliefs and practices in many parts of the world is an important shaper of what appears to be helpful for individuals. For example, although surveys suggest that the majority of Japanese and Chinese people will identify themselves as having no religion, belief in ghosts and the practice of ancestor worship will be used as a means of maintaining bonds which are necessary to achieve the notion of family wholeness essential to 'belonging' in these societies (Klass and Goss, 1999; Hsu et al, 2004). Similarly, Chinese people in the UK maintain westernised attitudes and lifestyles alongside preferring not to die at home because 'home' in the UK means a transient dwelling inhabited by the spirits of strangers; instead they engage in practices which symbolically return the spirit of the deceased to rest in the ancestral home (Payne et al, 2005). Further, the importance of religious and spiritual practices to many ethnic minority populations has contributed significantly to raising awareness of the significance of spirituality in bereavement more widely (Noppe and Noppe, 1999).

Second, different approaches to relationships and notions of relatedness dictate how the individual experience of bereavement pans out. If a good death is thought to be one in which harmony, reconciliation and (re)union is achieved with family, then any disruption to relationships, or failure to gather all family members together, will leave the bereaved at risk of guilt and anxiety. 'Relational connectedness' is a concept explored in Chinese literature. After the death, these notions also determine the way in which the bereaved must behave in terms of the relationship which is lost, relationships which remain and new relationships which may be formed. Thus the notion of 'continuing bonds' takes on a concrete reality in cultures where the dead are still required to exercise a responsible and supportive role with the living (Wallis, 2001). In such a context, the idea of 'letting go', as a sign of completion of grief, would be deeply disturbing.

The effects of widowhood have been particularly studied. It is a social state which varies considerably across cultures. For women, however, the existence of strong cultural norms, which predetermine acceptable behaviour, appear to be universal. The 'merry widow' in Anglo-Saxon culture excites a degree of social disapproval, and yet widows are also noted to be one of the groups most at risk of chronic grief. Silverman's research, which showed that white older North American widows are finding new outlets and creative energies, is thus both celebrated and the cause of some unease for overturning social assumptions (Silverman, 2004). Meanwhile, Elwert and Christakis (2006) found that black American widows do not experience the detrimental health effects, including increased mortality risk, usually attributed to widowhood, because their social context allows them to maintain the benefits normally associated with marriage. By contrast, in Taiwan, widows are seen as a pernicious influence disturbing the family balance and many are isolated in bereavement with their grief made more intense (Hsu et al, 2004).

Third, the relationship between culture and identity must be seen as a significant shaper of the experiencing and expression of grief, and identity must be understood as both a social and psychological phenomenon. Thus, for example, it is argued that suffering and dying are part of the black African-American identity arising from their history of slavery, and in consequence black Americans have high expectations that their mourning will be socially validated and facilitated

(Moore and Phillips, 1994). One can infer from this that any disappointment in the support available to a grieving person, or if their grief is disenfranchised, might be particularly problematic. On the other hand, anecdotal evidence in the UK suggests that younger British-born Afro-Caribbeans may experience difficulty precisely because they are charged to carry out the wishes of parents concerning traditional Jamaican rituals and styles of mourning. Adhering to the prescribed period and manner of Jewish mourning may be helpful to a person who is able to identify with the traditional Jewish understanding of life and death, but problematic to a person who does not and finds the practices alienating. The same can be said of any religion, and for the person whose cultural identity is inextricably entwined with a particular religion, feelings of alienation are likely to lead to complicated grief.

Fourth, cultural style also indicates the appropriate intervention. For example, in a culture which enjoys story-telling, opportunities to go over the story of the death and the relationship previously enjoyed may be informally available, and narrative therapies the most acceptable approach for the bereaved person who needs formal help. Encouragement to share emotion with strangers may be countercultural and unhelpful for someone else. At the same time, it should be remembered that having regard to cultural stereotypes ('excitable Frenchman', 'inscrutable Chinese') is not helpful when seeking to engage with the individual.

In outlining some broad principles, that might guide our understanding of grief across cultures, I am suggesting two things. First, that it is of critical importance to integrate the broad social and cultural context with the particular individual experience. Second, that while our knowledge base must be multicultural, understanding and respecting difference, our approach should be transcultural, that is, seeking out common reference points to further our understanding of the other person's grief. Finally, it should be remembered that although attitudes to death always uncover a degree of cultural stagnation, as, for example, seen in older Hong Kong Chinese in the UK as compared to their counterparts in Hong Kong (Payne et al, 2005), 'culture' itself is a dynamic concept which, when it comes to dying and bereavement in late modernity, encompasses both rapidly changing beliefs and practices and the maintenance of traditions.

Conclusion

In some ways this chapter is a contradiction. Whilst arguing that many of the criticisms of established theories stem from a crude application of a central idea without reflecting its nuances and caveats, I have provided a potted account of a huge range of theories from bereavement research, making selective use of the ideas of individual grief theorists. All the theories discussed, and particularly the work on complicated grief, are a great deal more sophisticated, with detailed sub-categorisation, than it has been possible to do justice to in this summary account; the reader is advised to follow up with further study any which they find particularly relevant. My mitigation, however, for such an overview is this:

should a description which large numbers of individuals, over time and still, intuitively feel is saying something of value, which resonates in some way with their own experience, be discarded? And if we are to benefit from this eclectic mix through enhanced understanding of a wider range of circumstances, there is merit in attempting to synthesise its distilled essence. Thus I have focused on those elements which appear to have enduring relevance, remembering that each, in application, must be individually, socially, culturally and philosophically contextualised according to the particular personality and circumstance. This, I suggest, is the best that practitioners can do in the day-to-day encounter. To do otherwise is to move to the one extreme of imposing a template, or the other of working atheoretically.

It is this mix which helps us to understand the negotiation of a pathway through grief, which takes place for the individual. However, despite the diverse theories now available and continuing development of new approaches, the popularity of the idea that there are common patterns to grieving, which can be constructed into models, remains). The focus also remains predominantly on the individual intra-psychic processes and consequent emotional response. Klass expresses disappointment that the controversy surrounding the introduction of continuing bonds theory to bereavement research has stayed in the realm of intra-psychic processes, whereas he sees its social and cultural components as at least as important (Klass, 2006).

Chapter Seven discusses contemporary forms of memorialisation, and the ways in which bereaved people use them to continue to connect with those who have died. It remains the case that the social dimension of bereavement research and sociological explanations of grief are much less developed than the psychological and psychiatric theories on which practitioners tend to draw. Although Kellehear pointed long ago to the need for social workers to have access to a sociology of death as well as the more familiar psychological models of grief (Kellehear, 1984), there is very little in the literature which seeks to fuse analysis of the social context of death with detailed psychological examination of the individual's experience of dying and bereavement, at least in a form which is helpful and relevant for the practitioner (Lloyd, 1992). There is even less which tackles with intellectual rigour the integration of theological and philosophical reflection with psychosocial approaches to dying and bereavement. This chapter and the preceding one have attempted to make some tenuous links, but there is much still to be done in developing an integrated approach to theoretically informed practice.

Key questions for practitioners

1. Which theories and approaches to bereavement and grief do I feel most comfortable with? What do they contribute to my practice?
2. Are there any with which I am uncomfortable? Why? What, if anything, could I take from these which might enhance my practice?
3. What issues are most challenging for me around bereavement and grief? Personally? In my work? What could grief theories contribute to helping me deal with these issues?
4. What do I see as the continuing gaps? In the theories? In my own work?

Notes

[1] See Fowler's *Modern English Usage* for the distinction between 'bereaved' and 'bereft'.

[2] Colin Murray Parkes makes the point that a psychiatric diagnosis is not made on the basis of the abnormality of the bereavement reaction but the degree of distress and disturbance (personal communication, January 2006).

[3] Colin Murray Parkes prefers to say that all deaths are special (personal communication). There is no attempt here to detract from the uniqueness of the individual death of whatever type.

FIVE

Dying in the twenty-first century

Introduction

Contemporary dying presents a series of questions for the dying person, their family and the professionals who attend them. These questions are embedded in complex ethical debates which have legal, medical, ideological, philosophical and religious ramifications. This situation arises from two features of modern life – the fact that medical advances allow us to control, to a great extent, both the manner and moment of death, and a concern for human rights, which constantly seeks to balance the rights of the individual with the wider interests of society. Woven through are a number of subsidiary issues which pose their own sets of questions. When is a person effectively dead? How do we determine capacity and incapacity and who should take 'life and death' decisions on behalf of a person deemed incapable of making their own? How do we determine quality of life? Are some lives more valuable than others when it comes to allocating resources or making treatment choices? Do a person's wishes and choices voiced at one point in time have currency when the situation changes? These and many more questions about the relationship between life and death face individuals and families in their personal lives and professionals in their daily work. All too frequently individuals find themselves surprisingly ill-prepared when confronted with a particular dilemma, despite increasing public debate, fuelled by some high-profile cases.

The ongoing demographic changes discussed in Chapter One have resulted in many of these issues seeming to crystallise in the care of older people. These are separately discussed in Chapter Six. However, they are by no means confined to dying in old age. Life support technologies are available to keep accident victims alive in states where once they would have died. Babies born prematurely are nurtured through survival into growth, but frequently with big questions hanging over their present and future quality of life. Sensitive issues surrounding organ donation and transplants have to be dealt with in situations of emotional stress and haste. Overall, the seemingly elastic boundary between life and death can make the enormity of a decision which is irreversible feel overwhelming. The shock of the cold finality of death is felt even when it is an event which was planned and prepared for.

For a long time it seemed that discussion of the ethical questions underlying and surrounding our technologically sophisticated medical and healthcare systems lagged behind the realities of practice. Not only did this leave patients and families adrift as they struggled with decisions put to them, it left doctors in particular, but other front-line healthcare professionals also, vulnerable in law and frequently feeling themselves to be on the horns of a dilemma, or personally compromised. What became evident is that the law is a blunt and mistaken instrument for resolving these dilemmas in practice and as a society we cannot afford to ignore them. Fortunately, while it cannot be claimed that we have arrived at all the answers, or indeed that there are any 'answers' in some situations, there is now an accumulating public and professional debate to inform deliberations and guide practice in the particular instance. Stimulated by the hospice movement, we also have some notion that there are better and worse ways to manage dying, and palliative care has pushed forward its approach to the former. The challenge is how to bring together philosophies, ideologies and pragmatics of care which contain within them contradictions.

Philosophies and ethos of care

We have seen in Chapter Two how the prevailing ethos in contemporary health and social care systems may be inimical to the development of quality care for people who are dying. The development of palliative care has been driven by a core philosophy which has to do with a focus on the whole person. This has been translated into objectives that now have international currency in both the developed and the developing worlds.

Hospice and palliative care

The World Health Organization (WHO) now defines palliative care as:

> an approach that improves the quality of life of patients and their families facing the problem associated with life-threatening illness, through the prevention and relief of suffering by means of early identification and impeccable assessment and treatment of pain and other problems, physical, psychosocial and spiritual. (World Health Organization, 2007).

The WHO statement goes on to stress the need for integrated care delivered by a multidisciplinary team and that palliative care strikes a balance between life-affirming and prolonging treatments and the acceptance of dying as a normal process.

The palliative care movement has grown out of the hospice movement, whose mission was originally driven forward through a philosophy of care which had four key points:

- attention to individual detail
- control of pain
- helping people to live until they die

- supporting the dying individual in a community of faith and hope (Saunders, 1990).

Hospices have stayed essentially true to this mission and all that it implies. For example, the St Christopher's hospice in South London (founded by Cicely Saunders) declares its mission as follows:

> St Christopher's exists to provide skilled and compassionate palliative care of the highest quality … St Christopher's care extends beyond the treatment of physical symptoms to consider the support, emotional, psychological, spiritual and social needs of our patients, their families, children, friends and carers. (www.stchristophers.org.uk)

This translates into an approach which aims to 'open up' dying. For staff this may involve confronting their own fears about dying in order that there are no emotional and psychological obstacles to continuing communication with the dying person. An emphasis on communication is a key aspect of hospice care and can be seen as a direct response to the cultures of 'closed awareness' (see Chapter Three) observed in hospitals in the mid-twentieth century, and still today in some instances (a recent Californian study found that families' experiences of communications with hospital doctors was 'one of interruption, inconclusion and marginalisation' [Russ and Kaufman, 2005, p 120]). There is concern that staff, family and friends should not 'cut the dying person off' prematurely, but stay in communication with them right to the end. As we shall see later in this chapter, there can be tensions between the objectives of staff to keep the patient fully engaged and in control of their life, and the wish of the dying person and their family for sedation. Although symptom and pain control are central tenets of hospice care, it is recognised that pain is not just physical, and that some symptoms are much more difficult to control than others. The notion of 'staying with the pain' alongside the dying person, including emotional, psychological and spiritual pain, is embedded in the hospice philosophy of care – 'total care for total pain'. So too is attention to individual wishes, such as a last trip, or hairdo, which are not a treatment necessity and may even be risky in terms of the patient's illness. They may, however, be important to the person's sense of wholeness and well-being and a valuable way of showing continuing investment in what remains of their life. Alongside this continuing maintenance of hope in the person, hospices acknowledge the losses experienced and anticipated by the dying person and their family and offer counselling and support beforehand and bereavement support after.

Such care is demanding of individual staff to offer and sustain at all times, and such a broad mission is increasingly difficult for voluntarily funded organisations to continue to pursue, especially when it cannot be justified in terms of easily measurable outcomes. It was shown in Chapter Two how the prevailing culture in health and social care is leading hospices to concentrate on the practical detail of palliative care. Increasingly, it is necessary to build the evidence base for aspects of hospice care which are not so easily demonstrated but which lie at its heart. For example, a large survey in the US of spouse survival rates post-bereavement suggested that the support offered through hospice care might attenuate the known mortality risk for bereaved spouses, particularly widows (Christakis, 2003). The case studies which form the basis for Chapter Eight, taken from current practice, illustrate some of these tensions, and at various points in this book there is discussion of how the hospice mission may at times be failing or distorted in some aspects. Nevertheless, hospices remain a potent force championing quality services and dignified care for people who are dying.

One way in which their role is changing in the shifting context of end-of-life care is analysed as 'managing the boundaries' between life and death. No longer do people just enter hospices in order to die, nor is the provision of hospice services confined to the building. Nevertheless, it is argued that hospices continue to create that liminal space in which people may make the transition from life to death (Froggatt, 1997). If this is to be facilitative it must not be undermined by poor transfers between services, where the energies of the dying person become dissipated in coping with discontinuities in care between different providers (Woods et al, 2006). As noted earlier, the move to make hospices into a fully integrated part of the health and social care network is a key element in the current agenda.

The extension of its philosophy and practice into all healthcare settings is currently the main thrust of palliative care, with calls for such care to be seen as a basic human right (Harding, 2006). The public health agenda which this implies – in terms of government policy, including ensuring universal availability of drugs for pain and symptom control, professional training, and raising public awareness – is being particularly promoted in countries hit by the HIV pandemic. However, there is continuing evidence that much still needs to be done in the developed world to make good palliative care available in hospitals, despite the setting up of specialist units. Until palliative care principles permeate the health and social care system, people at the end of life will remain vulnerable to experiencing insensitive care, ignorant of their total needs and the most appropriate ways of meeting them. Initiatives like the Liverpool Care Pathway for dying patients (Ellershaw et al, 1997) aim to disseminate the good practice of hospices and specialist palliative care units more widely, but its proponents acknowledge that transforming the 'culture' is difficult (Jack et al, 2005; Twomey et al, 2007). The House of Commons Health Committee, concluding its report on palliative care, emphasised the need to address social attitudes to death and dying if the culture in which dying takes place, and the care which is provided, are to change (HC Health Committee report, 2003–04).

Religion and spirituality

The hospice movement has emphasised spiritual care from the outset as part of a holistic approach which treats the whole person in their total context. Yet it is still claimed that much end-of-life care is 'spiritually barren' (Fetzer Institute, 2003). Across the range of palliative and end-of-life care, it is possible that both perspectives are true. Even within hospices, recognition of the existence of spiritual need and spiritual pain at the end of life is not matched by the same level of understanding about how to identify this need within the individual patient, or how to respond to it. This is despite the fact that a considerable amount of research has been conducted, in nursing in particular, aimed at trying to define spirituality and assess spiritual need.

The situation is complicated in western, secular societies by the fact that in the professional literature attention has been focused on distinguishing 'religion' from 'spirituality', a distinction which is often lost on lay people (McSherry, 2007). Lay people do, however, recognise that facing death causes most people to grapple with some of the 'bigger questions', although the extent to which these are significant and how big the question is, will vary enormously (Lloyd, 1997). Moss suggests that spirituality is 'what we do to give expression to our chosen world view' (Moss, 2005, p 60), which places it into a wider frame than definitions such as the search for meaning which may have little to distinguish them from humanistic counselling (Holloway, 2007) or what others might term social or psychological needs (Kellehear, 2000). Kellehear distinguishes 'situational', 'moral and biographical' and 'religious' needs as commonly featuring in discussions of spirituality in contemporary palliative care, observing, however, that each of the two former categories may be overlaid with 'religious desire' in the individual. Situational needs, he suggests, are concerned with meaning and purpose, moral and biographical needs are largely relational and concerned with harmony and reconciliation, whereas religious needs address all these through belief in a divine entity and purpose.

The secular caring professions have been concerned to distance themselves from any association with institutional religion in their interest in spirituality, the suggestion appearing to be that in so doing they would alienate non-religious persons who nevertheless have spiritual needs – and the common observation of nurses in palliative care, who perhaps spend the most time directly with the dying person, is that 'everyone' has spiritual needs. Palliative care professionals in northern Europe and Australasia have tended to pay little more than lip-service to their role in this less defined spiritual care. In southern Europe there may be strong identification with the religious foundation of the hospice with 'spiritual care' delivered through this medium and the distinction between religion and spirituality may be of no importance. Only the US, generally recognised to be a much more religious society than the UK or other northern European countries, has seen the active development of spiritual care functions among secular professionals, with the emergence of what some have dubbed 'surrogate chaplains' (Paley, 2007).

This 'spiritual but not religious' distinction belongs to the mainstream 'post-Christian' cultures of the west. It exists alongside a growing interest in palliative care in facilitating the religious requirements of 'other' religions, particularly those of ethnic minority families. This mostly takes the form of describing the rituals and sacraments important in the particular faith and making suggestions about how palliative care professionals can work alongside the family and their religious adviser. For example, emphasis is placed on the importance for Buddhists of a peaceful environment at the point of death, in which the 'transfer of consciousness' may take place with the dying person's sense of well-being enhanced as they focus on their death and rebirth. This suggests many things for the behaviour of healthcare professionals in the days and hours leading up to the death and immediately after death has occurred. For example, they should minimise disturbances, such as routine checks and avoid unnecessary noise, such as pagers going off whilst attending to the patient. The body should be left in place for as long as possible after the death (Dinh et al, 2000; Barham, 2003; Smith-Stoner, 2005).

Belief in karma, that one's deeds in one existence determine the state into which one is reborn, implies that all should be done for the Hindu to make the death 'good', since past misdeeds may be redeemed through the mode of dying. For some Hindus this may include the patient endurance of suffering, pain relief not being requested; the imparting of wisdom to surviving members of the family (katha); and the avoidance of food and drink so as to purify the body and avoid contaminating symptoms such as incontinence (Gatrad et al, 2003). Being in a state of preparedness is essential and the completion of social, psychological and emotional tasks – such as setting one's affairs in order, saying goodbye to relatives – belong to this spiritual preparation. Where some aspect of the death is 'bad karma', it is the sacred duty of relatives to try to undo its effects through rituals and good deeds (Firth, 2005). Thus, healthcare practice which obstructs or denies the opportunity for the Hindu patient to have their own 'good death' may have lasting implications for the family. In Islam, a number of detailed rituals are proscribed (Ross, 2001). These centre around beliefs about the relationship between the body and spirit, and the soul as the unique mix of both in each individual. In death, the soul is released from the body to commence its passage into the spiritual realm. It is important not to violate the body in any way as this may lead to contamination of the soul, but organ harvesting is allowed once death has occurred, since the preservation of life is a sacred goal. The Jewish tradition, meanwhile, places greater emphasis on the obligation to heal, which implies both that the patient should cooperate with medical procedures advised by their doctor, and that relatives, friends and healthcare providers should attend to the social, emotional and spiritual needs of the person who is dying. Creating a community in which the individual's dying might take place, and avoiding isolating the patient if at all possible, should therefore be the objective of good palliative care (Dorff, 2005).

The point that is in danger of being lost when the focus is on the rites and rituals of a particular religious tradition is that for committed adherents of any religious faith – including Christians – death is an event of deep spiritual significance and dying is imbued with spiritual meaning. These meanings may be experienced positively or negatively, and every professional, not just the chaplain or religious adviser, contributes to that experience by their attitudes and behaviour. The existence of spiritual pain and existential distress or despair are beginning to be recognised as significant, as much for the religious person as for the non-religious (Parker, 2004). Parker describes the core phenomena of existential distress as hopelessness, helplessness, powerlessness, loss of a sense of control and a sense of meaninglessness. Spiritual pain, however, may further personal growth and ultimately be an enriching experience (Burton, 2004).

This may affect the carer of someone who is dying as much as the dying person. A study in America described informal carers as accompanying the dying person 'through the existential challenges of the transition to the unknown' (Pearce et al, 2006, p 755*)*. This study found that where their spiritual experience was a positive resource on which to draw it contributed to feeling that they could bear the pain and burden of their situation and sometimes derive spiritual enrichment from it. Where they experienced their situation as being abandoned or punished by God, or implying that God was powerless, however, they were more likely to find their situation burdensome and sometimes unbearable. In a survey of hospital social workers and chaplains which I undertook in the early 1990s, 86 per cent said that they recognised spiritual pain in the dying and bereaved people they worked with but the social workers as a whole did not see themselves as having any part to play in spiritual care (Lloyd, 1997).

The existence of untreated depression is a significant factor to be taken into account in any end-of-life decision making. However, there is a balance to be achieved between appropriate psychiatric care and seeking to medicalise something – existential despair – which defies medical solution (Parker, 2004). An alternative is to see connecting with the spiritual meanings of the other person as an essential part of sensitive care, regardless of the specific belief position of the individual patient, relative or worker. Such an approach is transcultural, in that it seeks to access the strengths and resources both within the other person and within a tradition which has meaning for them (Holloway, 2006a).

The good death

At the heart of palliative care a concept has developed which has come to be referred to as 'the good death'. The origins of the term are twofold. First, as is often pointed out in discussions of euthanasia, the Greek translates as 'good death', literally meaning dying 'well' or painlessly. However, as Kellehear (1990) has pointed out, there is also another Greek word used to describe a good death, in which the emphasis is on dying according to a socially acceptable and prescribed pattern. The 'art of dying well' pre-dates the modern articulation and historically was built around some quite opposite values, including the value of suffering and the rewards of sainthood (Walters, 2004). In its reaction against the common experiences of dying in the modern, impersonal hospital, geared to cure rather than care, the hospice movement took the notion of pain relief and comfortable dying and combined it with social, psychological and spiritual objectives to arrive at a model for dying which was 'good'. Thus the notion of the 'good death' which has gained widespread currency in contemporary palliative care has accommodated both meanings in the original Greek through a reaction against all that was bad about modern dying. This may be one reason why ideas of good and bad dying have become somewhat stylised among healthcare professionals, with all the problems that imposing a 'right way' to die may have in terms of responding to individual patient need (Lloyd, 1995; Jones and Willis, 2003; Walters, 2004). Furthermore, this idealised picture may belong more to palliative care than to the wider society, since few studies have been undertaken which actually gathered the views of patients and their families (McNamara et al, 1994; Mak and Clinton, 1999). Payne et al (1996) found that while staff tended to pursue a policy of 'open awareness', encouraging a situation in which the patient was conscious and in control of their dying, patients themselves were most concerned about a pain-free death.

Nevertheless, by the early 1990s a consensus had emerged in the literature and in healthcare practice about what constituted 'the good death'. There are a number of elements which appear to have international and cross-cultural acceptance:

- to die at peace, with one's affairs in order;
- to be free from pain;
- to die in a place of one's choosing;
- to be surrounded by and reconciled with loved ones;
- to be treated with respect and afforded dignity.

These were elaborated upon in 1999 in the UK by an Age Concern study group, which produced twelve principles:

1. to know when death is coming, and to understand what can be expected;
2. to be able to retain control of what happens;
3. to be afforded dignity and privacy;
4. to have control over pain relief and other symptom control;
5. to have choice and control over where death occurs (at home or elsewhere);
6. to have access to information and expertise of whatever kind is necessary;
7. to have access to any spiritual or emotional support required;
8. to have access to hospice care in any location, not only in hospital;
9. to have control over who is present and who shares the end;
10. to be able to issue advance directives which ensure wishes are respected;
11. to have time to say goodbye, and control over other aspects of timing;
12. to be able to leave when it is time to go, and not to have life prolonged pointlessly (Debate of the Age Health and Care Study Group, 1999).

The flurry of responses which appeared in the pages of the *British Medical Journal* (*BMJ*) after it published these principles underlined the fact that, while few disagreed with these principles as aims, we have rather less control over death than they might appear to suggest. A debate in the *BMJ* three years later also argued that undue weight is placed on some aspects of care and others, such as mental health needs and psychological care, are ignored (Prigerson et al, 2003). The notion of personhood, discussed in Chapter Three under the category of 'personal death', is at the heart of the good death but becomes implicit rather than explicit the more criteria are defined. These discussions illustrate the complexity of applying, in practice, those key objectives of contemporary health and social care of person-centred care which affords dignity, choice and control to the individual.

Bradbury asks, 'For whom is a death good?', and argues that we have multiple representations in our society of both good and bad deaths and contemporary ideas do not necessarily accord with those of previous generations (Bradbury, 2001, p 59). For example, when infant and child mortality rates were high, these deaths could be deemed 'natural' by comparison with contemporary developed societies where death of a child is viewed as 'untimely'. This did not mean that such deaths were seen as 'good', or as the preferred outcome. The same can be said of deaths of children in the developing world, where aid workers and television images testify to the grief of parents at the loss of every child, even though they might struggle to feed and care for them, and deaths of children are shockingly commonplace. Bradbury distinguishes three types of good death: the sacred, the medicalised and the natural. The sacred is located in a belief system which sees death as the gateway to a better existence; the medicalised is one which is controlled through medical intervention; the natural is one which occurs without such intervention and, according to Bradbury, unexpectedly – for example, dying in one's sleep. Another very common contemporary idea is that a natural death is one which occurs when one has reached the end of one's natural lifespan. Bad deaths, by definition, occur when the opposite circumstance prevails. So, bad ways to die are when the individual takes himself or herself out of the hands of God by committing suicide; or evil appears to prevail as in murder; or pain and distressing symptoms are not well controlled; or the death is in some way untimely, occurring as a result of accident or there is 'unfinished business' and/or the individual is unable to prepare.

Bradbury touches on the fact that the complexities of contemporary dying mean that the types tend to get mixed up. It is worth pursuing this if we are to better understand and respond to the needs of diverse people and situations. First, since almost all deaths are medicalised to some degree and, as the next section makes clear, significant and multiple ethical issues are raised by the possibilities created by medical intervention, it is most likely to be the accommodation reached between medicalised death and the beliefs about death and dying held by the individual and family that will determine whether or not this is a good death for them. So, for example, someone who wishes for a 'natural' death in their sleep may adjust this concept to include terminal sedation. Someone with strong religious faith, who believes that life and death are in the hands of God, may be grateful for the best of medical intervention but accommodate suffering and untimely death as part of 'God's plan'. I vividly recall a Muslim woman whose baby had been stillborn, being uncomprehending of the suggestion that it might help her to talk about her feelings, because her baby's death had been 'Allah's will'. A narrative may be constructed which sees the death as good because it touched the lives of others, carrying within it creative and regenerative possibilities for other people (Maudlin, 2001); because learning to accept rather than control death is spiritually transforming (Peterson, 2000; Crosby, 2004); because the baby born with a congenital disorder had reached the end of her natural lifespan and was ready to die (Guthrie, 2000). This mother reflects, from a non-religious position, a number of these ways of concluding that her baby had died a good death:

> 'In this whole process of life and death for *baby* it just wasn't meant to be … I feel that she was actually given to us for a reason, but that she was actually only meant to live for ten and a half months, but in that time, the effect she had, not just on us, but on other people was, well, astounding.' (Lloyd, 1996, p 302)

These ways of understanding the good death expand the concept from the physical process of dying and the moment of death. It is possible that they can accommodate features of 'bad' deaths – such as symptoms which cannot be well controlled – because meaning is ascribed to and emphasis placed on other aspects. Within the established model of the good death, delivered through good palliative care, such deaths are hard for patients and staff to accommodate, because both may have expectations which are disappointed. Lawton (1998) in an ethnographic study of hospice care, observed that increasingly hospices may be used to accommodate those patients whose symptoms are such that they cannot be contained in community palliative care. Her study suggested that this 'dirty dying' transgresses all the boundaries which our vision of 'dying well' has erected, leading to staff separating these patients off from others for whom they can better achieve a good death. If this picture were to become widespread – and there are some suggestions that it is (Bowling, 2003; Kalbag, 2003) – we should have a situation in which, ironically, hospices are contributing to the sequestration of death, not only within the wider society, but also within themselves.

There are further problems in promoting this idealised type of the good death. It belongs to a western philosophical model which gives primary emphasis to the individual and their medical care. The uncritical application of the value of autonomy is problematic. By definition, the person who is near death must rely on someone else to maintain control according to their wishes on their behalf. Dying with dignity is as much about having one's vulnerability respected as it is about exercising autonomy. Grogono (2003) advocates appointing an 'amicus mortis', a trusted friend or relative, but not everyone has such a person available. Second, it has taken repeated efforts to remind healthcare providers that respect for different cultural and religious practices as well as belief systems has to underpin this medical care and affect its mode of delivery (Neuberger, 2003). Walter suggests that different models of the good death emanate from different societal and cultural norms, but that these in turn relate to three factors; the extent of secularisation; the extent of individualism; and the length of time it takes to die (Walter, 2003). Campione argues that in Italy religious, materialistic-biological and 'personalistic' concepts of the good death are intertwined – not necessarily in each individual death, but in the social context in which dying is managed (Campione, 2004).

We have as yet little empirical evidence to test Walter's assertion. What we have, suggests a surprising degree of consensus concerning core elements across quite different societies. For example, a study in Uganda identified the desire to die at home, to be free from pain and other distressing symptoms, to experience no stigma (this appears to relate to the high levels of death through HIV/AIDS), to be at peace and to retain a degree of autonomy whilst having one's needs met (Kikule, 2003). Two studies of Chinese people, one undertaken in Hong Kong and the other in the UK, suggested that pain and symptom control and a physically 'comfortable' death were a priority as well as not being a burden on family; this led in the UK to a preference for not dying at home. However, relational aspects were also emphasised – knowing that one's family relationships were intact, with children and grandchildren established and happy, and to have them around the bedside; knowing that one had completed one's business in life and the spirit could be released peacefully (Quality Evaluation Centre, City University of Hong Kong, unpublished survey results; Payne et al, 2005). However, these summary findings tell us little about what may in practice be crucial differences and important contributory factors to a good or bad death. For example, Walter cites the example of Hindus' wish to die lying on the floor, in accordance with their beliefs, and not liking to ask for this to be facilitated in western medical care; food is both medicine and comfort in Chinese culture and it is important for family members to provide certain foods for the sick and dying person; Chinese migrants prefer not to die at home because, unlike the ancestral home, 'home' is a transitory abode inhabited by the spirits of strangers; African languages and aboriginal peoples do not distinguish between 'secular' and 'religious' and spiritual care is an assumed part of dying well. The complex web of cultural assumptions and imperatives which may lead to a particular individual death being deemed 'good' is illustrated by the story told by Elizabeth Grant of a woman dying of cancer in sub-Saharan Africa. Paradoxically to the western mind, this woman expressed the wish to die when in hospital with her pain controlled and receiving good physical care, where earlier, experiencing terrible pain and deprivations at home, she had declared herself content to rest on God's timing (Grant, 2003).

What is clear is that the notion of the good death has to expand to deal with the fact that the majority of contemporary deaths in the developed world take place over a period of time, as people live with life-threatening illness or slow degenerative conditions. Thus, the focus is gradually shifting from the original model of hospice and palliative care towards end-of-life care which aims to provide quality for individuals in the 'dying phase' of life.

End-of-life-care

Evidence of the increasing numbers of people dying from a range of life-threatening conditions, particularly in old age, is widening the remit of care for the dying. Health and social care is beginning to recognise that good care for many people with chronic, disabling conditions is also good end-of-life care, and the proven tenets of palliative care, developed in the main around cancer patients, should be transferred into other care settings.

The policy context and initiatives for this were discussed in Chapter Two. At the heart of this initiative is to increase choice about their care for all people at the end of life and to ensure that those choices are respected wherever possible (Institute of Medicine, 2001; NHS, 2006). This is in the light of information that most people do not die at home even though just over half in the UK, US and Australia are reported as expressing the wish to do so (Fried et al, 1998; Higginson et al, 1998). The picture is actually rather more nuanced than these figures would suggest and the complexities surrounding the making and sustaining of choices are discussed in Chapter Six.

Nevertheless, there is growing interest in the making and implementing of choices concerning end-of-life care and the tools which might be available to assist with this. Behind this lies the question of incapacity, that in the event of becoming incapable of making and/or expressing their views, individuals may wish to make them known in advance of that situation. Not unnaturally, given that people are living longer but with increasing physical and mental debility, much of the debate among care providers about the facilitation and implementation of such expressions relates to older people. The focus of attention here tends to be on directives to withhold treatment (including the wish not to be resuscitated), although more recent emphases are on a positive care planning approach. The issues and evidence in the context of older people's care are discussed in Chapter Six. The high-profile cases, raised periodically in the media, tend to feature younger adults with seriously debilitating, degenerative diseases, who may wish to put in place a request for physician-assisted suicide and to identify the point at which they wish this to be activated. Where this challenges the legal position in a particular country, or moves into a 'grey area', the case is taken out of the patient and healthcare professional arena and into the courts.

The legal status of these tools varies from country to country. However, the general drift is as follows for the UK:

- *Advance directives or living wills*: both terms are currently in use. These documents allow the individual to express their wishes about specific medical interventions, commonly concerning 'do not resuscitate' (DNR) orders and artificial hydration or nutrition. They may be combined with designating 'power of attorney' to someone else to make, or instigate, these decisions for the person completing the original directive.

- *Enduring power of attorney*: under legislation in the UK about to be implemented, power of attorney is extended from financial and property matters to cover all aspects of the health and social care of a person deemed 'incapable' of making decisions for themselves.
- *Advance care planning*: this is carried out between the service user and the care provider(s). It is likely to become a crucial part of long-term care provision in the twenty-first century as a means of facilitating user choice.

The gathering of evidence concerning the use of such measures is so far in its early stages and the focus has tended to be on the care of older people and limited to healthcare directives. This evidence specific to older people is considered in the next chapter. The wider use of more holistic advance care planning procedures is still in its infancy. Young adults with life-threatening illnesses, for example, have been found to have little knowledge of advance directives or planning (Pendergast, 2001). However, some factors can be highlighted generally which have relevance for the management of dying in the community.

Making the point that most advance care planning takes place far too late and often in the hospital or office, thus effectively excluding seriously ill people and their relatives from playing an active part in the planning process, an American study piloted and evaluated the use of social worker-facilitated discussions in the home with people in receipt of home care, of whom 29 per cent were under 65; each had been diagnosed as having a life-threatening illness with a life expectancy of up to two years. A key goal of the intervention was to honour service user wishes concerning the site of their end-of-life care; this was achieved in the majority of cases, with 70 per cent of those who died during the study period being cared for at home as they had wished. The researchers highlight two important factors contributing to this success: emphasis was on the communicative process between worker and service user, rather than the exercise of patient autonomy; and the intervention was offered to people identified by the community nurse, who understood their individual history, circumstances and illness progression.

Haley et al (2002) also emphasise the importance of advance care planning taking place within the family and intimate relationships. They make the point that two groups are particularly vulnerable to inappropriate decision making and receiving unwanted care if the present emphasis on individual autonomy and legal status continues to override other considerations. Ethnic minority groups may feel their cultural sensitivities, including how decisions are taken within the family, are ignored. Partners without legal status (such as is frequently the case in same-sex partnerships) may be excluded, despite the fact that they may be intimately involved in care-giving in the home and their emotional investment greater than that of other persons who might be consulted as 'next of kin'.

A final point about advance directives and living wills is that, unlike advance care planning, they are often located in controversial and ethically disputed terrains. They may also involve established and relatively uncontentious procedures (except for some religious groups) such as organ donation, where the individual opts to forgo life-prolonging treatment and choose to donate organs. Advance directives are in themselves opposed by some religious groups on the grounds of individuals attempting a degree of control which does not belong to them, either in terms of their own life or in relation to the actions of others (O'Connor, 2005). These are the questions to which we now turn.

Euthanasia and assisted dying

In contrast to the palliative care approach which seeks to maintain and sustain the dying person as comfortably as possible at the end of life, a number of interventions have emerged where the objective is to hasten or bring about the person's death. These may involve the person alone, the person assisted by a friend or relative, a doctor acting on the wishes of the patient or the wishes of next of kin where the person themselves is incapable of giving consent, or, more rarely, the medical team acting on their professional judgement after seeking an external ruling on the matter. Both the legal position and extent to which these options are practised are unclear and vary between countries. Switzerland is credited with having been the first state, since 1942, to allow assisted suicide, provided that the helpers are 'disinterested' persons, although it is suggested that relatives of seriously ill patients are now asked to sanction euthanasia (Gardner, 2003). Significant attempts have been made in the western world in the last decade to legislate for the circumstances, constraints and procedures under which such practices might be carried out: the 1996 Rights of the Terminally Ill Amendment Act, Northern Territory, Australia; the Oregon Death with Dignity Act; the legalising of euthanasia and physician-assisted suicide (PAS) in Holland in 2002; the legalising of euthanasia by doctors but not PAS in Belgium in 2002. Evidence of actual practice is increasingly emerging and there are recent important legal initiatives, such as the Joffe 'assisted dying' Bill in the UK.

A good place to start in tackling this subject is to define the terminology. Problems arise in dissecting the issues when terms are used to mean different practices. The UK House of Lords report (HL, 1993–94) points out how the use of some terms, such as 'passive euthanasia', has been misleading and arrives at the following definitions:

- *euthanasia* – originally meaning a gentle and easy death, now used to mean a deliberate intervention to end a life where the patient's condition is terminal and their suffering 'intractable';
- *withdrawing treatment; not initiating treatment; treatment-limiting decision* – preferred to 'passive euthanasia' and used to refer to a medical decision not to give treatment necessary for the prolonging of life;
- *double effect* – the administration of treatment to relieve pain or severe distress where the likely consequence is that it will hasten death;
- *voluntary euthanasia* – brought about where the patient requests their own death;

- *non-voluntary euthanasia* – where the patient does not have the capacity to understand what euthanasia means and therefore to either request it or withhold consent;
- *involuntary euthanasia* – where life is terminated for someone who does have the capacity to make a request or give consent but has not actually done so;
- *assisted suicide* – where someone capable of making the decision to end their life desires this but is physically unable to bring about their death without assistance;
- *physician-assisted suicide* – which occurs when that help is given by a doctor, for example providing a lethal dose of a drug;
- *terminal illness*[1]– a progressive illness which will inevitably result in death within a short period of time;
- *irreversible condition* – a condition which is not progressive, often present at birth, and does not necessarily lead to death;
- *chronic progressive disease* – where deterioration is inevitable but may not of itself bring on death;
- *persistent vegetative state* – absence of cognitive, behavioural, verbal, or purposive motor responses over a period of not less than 12 months, with no evidence of other voluntary motor activity.

Certainly it is euthanasia which is the word most likely to raise public interest and rouse passions, although as can be seen from the above definitions, specific interventions may seem to merge in practice (for example, physician-assisted suicide and voluntary euthanasia, despite the fact that the amended Joffe Bill insists that a clear distinction must be drawn between them). Phrases such as the 'right to die' have become sloganised and concepts such as 'dignity in dying' appropriated by opposing camps. The issues are discussed in terms of three debates (although the arguments similarly merge): the moral-ethical debate; religion and euthanasia; and palliative care and euthanasia.

The moral-ethical debate

The philosophical case for euthanasia stems from a privileging of the principle of autonomy, that an individual has an absolute right to determine that they wish to die. This can be suicide at any point in life or voluntary euthanasia when the suffering in one's life becomes intolerable or it is anticipated that it will become so. More recent articulations of the 'right to die' add to it the 'responsibility to die'. From a philosophical standpoint this will be limited to a narrow range of specific situations in which one's death is imperative in order to serve the greater good, even that the greater good may be jeopardised otherwise. The example often cited is the suicide of a captured soldier lest he reveal secrets under torture which may lead to the deaths of many others. There are also vestiges of this thinking in 'hero' stories where one person sacrifices him/herself in order to make it more likely that others will survive (for example, an injured member of a climbing expedition party). While some utilitarian philosophers do extend this principle to a moral obligation to remove oneself when one's continuing existence is too much of a burden on society, others are much more cautious about the responsibilities and obligations surrounding the question of interconnectedness, pointing out that the individual who contemplates ending their life also has responsibility for the potential distress this may cause their loved ones (Nuyen, 2000). This is especially the case where the relative or friend is asked to assist in the act bringing about the death or in creating the circumstances in which it might take place.

The philosophical case 'for' is countered by a philosophical case against – although Nuyen suggests that the case against has become remarkably muted, the question of to what extent euthanasia should be legalised and institutionalised having taken over (Nuyen, 2000). Principally, the privileging of individual autonomy is challenged. Williams asks why autonomy should carry any more weight than the principle of the sanctity of life, and suggests that to give autonomy such moral authority infers that society is composed wholly of consenting adults (Williams, 1996). However, Harris takes issue with a privileging of the sanctity of life which fails to distinguish between existence, per se, and the lives of persons. Harris believes the case for euthanasia rests on respect for individuals who embody personhood, which he describes as a critical appreciation of one's own existence. If such a person wishes to die, Harris believes, it is both an arrogance and a tyranny to frustrate that desire (Harris, 1995).

However, others argue that if the case for euthanasia rests ultimately on the individual's right to choose to die, then there is no case for those people who have lost the capacity to exercise that choice, whatever their condition (Finnis, 1995). The case against is filled out by discussion of the question of intent, where the argument is put forward that the *moral* argument against euthanasia as a form of 'intentional killing' does not extend to the use of drugs where death occurs as an unintentional, although likely, side effect, or the declining of life-prolonging treatment because its impact is, in itself, undesirable. However, it does extend to the withdrawal of treatment or care, with the intent to bring about death (Finnis, 1995). Harris argues that there is no moral argument against such actions where personhood has been lost, suggesting that were an individual in a persistent vegetative state to have earlier completed an advance directive outlining their wish to be kept 'alive' whatever their condition, this would have no moral precedence over other 'critical interests' – including that health service resources might be put to better use.

A significant angle within the philosophical debate concerns the ethical obligations of doctors. The Hippocratic oath is usually taken as the starting point, with there being general agreement that doctors have a duty to sustain life and refrain from intentional killing. However, it is argued that both the particulars of individual cases (Meilaender, 2005) and the presence of competing moral duties – such as to relieve suffering – lead to the conclusion that no one moral position can be taken to be absolute or to always override another (Seay, 2005). From this standpoint there is no reason to try and distinguish between letting someone die, physician-assisted suicide, or double effect (Huxtable, 2004), because each privileges a different moral duty – refraining from intentional killing, the ending of suffering, or the relief of suffering such that death is likely. Indeed, Frey (2005) argues that it is the moral context of how we see the alternative – for example, allowing this child in this condition to die – which determines the morality of the action (or inaction). Despite the apparently irreconcilable philosophical positions on euthanasia, Meilaender (2005) argues that there is considerable consensus on some critical starting points when it comes to the application of moral ethics:

- We do not believe that 'biological life' must be preserved at all costs.
- We combine adherence to first principles with forming judgements about particular cases.
- Each life is of equal value and our aim should be to preserve rather than to end it.
- Respect for human life implies caring for the individual life in such a way as to allow that there may be a greater good than the continuation of that life in some circumstances.

Religion and euthanasia

The straightforward religious position, as represented by all the world's major religions, is that it is not for human beings to decide the moment of their own, or another's, death. This does not mean that compassion should not be shown for human suffering, including the mental and spiritual anguish of the person who takes their own life for whatever reason. This principle did, however, lie behind the ruling until 1961 in the UK that persons who had committed suicide could not be interred in consecrated ground. Conscientious objectors who refuse to fight in war on religious grounds are applying the same principle. The majority position in the Christian and Muslim religions, however, is that a just war and/or a soldier's duty are special circumstances in which other principles take precedence. Euthanasia, on the other hand, is generally considered wrong by religious thinkers. The positions of the major faiths were summarised thus in *USA Today* following the passing of the Oregon Death with Dignity Act:

> CATHOLIC: 'We are encouraged, if our end is to be loving, to examine how can we do that best. I don't love someone best by saying, "There are no possibilities for you, no hope or meaning …" Who am I to say that?' – the Rev. Kevin Fitzgerald.
>
> PROTESTANT: 'The New Testament teaches that we are to model ourselves on Christ. I'm not really to live for myself. I'm to live for the glory of God and the life of others' – bioethicist C. Ben Mitchell.
>
> JEWISH: 'You are given a self when you are born, but you can't willfully destroy it. You can refuse to prolong dying or to deepen the pain with

> interventions. But (suicide) ends all possibility of human flourishing' – Laurie Zoloth, medical ethics professor.
>
> MUSLIM: 'Islam rules (suicide) out. The trend is to accept your destiny as God-given destiny. Suffering is not regarded as evil, and there is faith that God … helps people to endure pain and suffering' – Abdulaziz Sachedina, religion professor.
>
> BUDDHIST: 'There are famous Buddhists in history who have committed suicide, but by far most Buddhist ethicists would say this is unacceptable. A doctor who assists someone in dying is called the "knife-bringer"' – Paul Numrich, author of *The Buddhist Tradition: Religious Beliefs and Healthcare Decisions.*
>
> HINDU: 'You and I cannot take our lives into our own hands. It is regarded as a form of ego. This ego keeps you in bondage in the cycle of reincarnation' – S. Cromwell Crawford, author of *Hindu Bioethics for the 21st Century.*
>
> (*USA Today*, 5 October 2005)

However, there is something of a debate around suffering, compassion and healing through death. A widely held view is that medical interventions which are no longer bringing any benefit but merely prolonging life may be withdrawn or withheld, but aggressive use of painkillers or other deliberate acts to bring about death are wrong (Gushee, 2004). The distinction is made in Catholic theology between impermissible intended consequences and those which are permissible because while the consequences are not intended they can be foreseen (the doctrine of 'double effect'). There are four conditions imposed: the action itself must not be inherently wrong (for example, administering analgesics); the intention must be to produce the good effect (for example, the drugs are administered for the relief of pain); the good effect must not be brought about via the bad effect (for example, pain should be relieved before and without death occurring); the good effect must outweigh the bad (for example, relief of suffering was the primary outcome). Some take this line further and argue that resisting death when one's time has come (including through disease) is also wrong (Hatzinikolaou, 2003); indeed death should be welcomed and seen as the healer (Grad, 1980).

Mohrmann, as a paediatrician and medical ethicist, argues that religion has paid scant attention to children as beings and hence to their rights and our responsibilities towards them. She suggests that these can only be discharged when seen in the context also of the needs of those who care for, and about, children. Thus, the suffering of parents must also be taken into account when determining benefit of treatments, particularly where the benefits are uncertain (Mohrmann, 2006).

Islamic guidance for healthcare professionals is connected to the principle of beneficence, whereby positive actions to prevent or remove what is bad or harmful and to promote what is good or beneficial are required; the direct termination of life, however, must be left in the hands of Allah (Rassool, 2004). Within Chinese culture, there is agreement between Confucianism, Buddhism and Taoism that life should be cherished as a natural process but not be attached to; adherents are likely to be opposed to active euthanasia but comfortable with the notion of 'letting die', the natural process therefore taking over (Chong and Fok, 2005). In Israel, the context is complex, combining both the Jewish Orthodox tradition with a political context which favours communitarianism over individual autonomy and is sharply mindful of its twentieth-century history at the hands of the Nazis. The Israeli Patient Rights Law (1996) requires all cases of 'informed refusal' of medical treatment to be referred to an ethics committee in which the religious interest may be outweighed by others (Leichtentritt, 2002).

Palliative care and euthanasia

One of the most intense debates has been between advocates of euthanasia and palliative care specialists. The position originally taken by the latter was that good palliative care, with adequate relief of pain and other distressing symptoms, more or less obviates the demand for euthanasia – or, to put it another way, that the policy emphasis should be on making good palliative care available and accessible to all, rather than looking to legislate for euthanasia. However, it is now recognised that some palliative care patients do nevertheless request a hastening of their death and that doctors in palliative care face the dilemma over double treatment effect as much as elsewhere.

In 2001, the European Association for Palliative Care (EAPC) established a Task Group to advise them on euthanasia and physician-assisted suicide. The Task Group published a position paper (Materstvedt et al, 2003) alongside 55 responses from academics, clinicians, practitioners and researchers from 32 different countries. This published debate represents the most significant airing of the issues to date. One of the important things it establishes is that the musings of philosophers about definitions, moral boundaries and moral duties are not simply abstract conceptualisations; they are reflected in the thinking of clinicians and practitioners as they struggle with real-life dilemmas (Campbell and Huxtable, 2003). The position paper itself is succinct and acknowledges the deeply divided views while generally rejecting voluntary euthanasia (on which it focuses) as being able to sit alongside palliative care. There is some empirical evidence for this view: a New York study showed that healthcare professionals in a cancer centre who were more inclined towards assisted suicide had correspondingly less knowledge about symptom management (Portenoy et al, 1997). However, evidence from the Netherlands about the effect of provision for euthanasia on palliative care practice is said to be contradictory (Hurst and Mauron, 2006).

In an editorial reviewing both the EAPC Task Force paper and responses to it, Campbell and Huxtable conclude that both the theoretical underpinnings for arriving at a particular conclusion on euthanasia, and evidence about the effects on palliative care of new legislation, require considerably more investigation.

Although not highlighted by the editorial, important points about the cultural context of palliative care, including the extent to which there is a culture in which diagnosis and care are discussed with the patient and/or the family, are made by contributors. Greater clarity of definition and consensus concerning the use of these definitions are highlighted as essential. In particular, without open discussion of the relationship between motivation and intent, of patient competence and incompetence, and of the determining of a 'terminal' condition and the notion of 'mercy killing', clinicians and practitioners in palliative care settings will continue to be dogged by uncertainty and ambiguity. A useful contribution to this clarification exercise is contributed in a paper from Switzerland, which argues for a number of values held in common by advocates of voluntary euthanasia (VE) and assisted suicide (AS), and palliative care. Four shared underpinning values are identified: the importance of reducing suffering; a concern to maintain a focus on the dying *person* rather than biological entity; the importance of the patient retaining some control at the end of life; an acceptance that death is not always the worst thing to happen (Hurst and Mauron, 2006). However, as the authors point out, it is how these values are understood in practice where differences remain and need further exploration. For example, compassion is interpreted by palliative care to mean 'staying with' the patient's pain (understood holistically) even as one seeks to relieve it, whereas advocates of VE/AS view this as itself the compassionate act. They acknowledge that some positions, such as whether the value of individual autonomy ever overrides the principle of not ending human life, may be irreconcilable. So too may the conflict between the physician's right to autonomy and the duty of care which respects the patient's right to make decisions about their own quality of life.

Clearly, the legal position in most countries makes it difficult to gather empirical evidence, and conclusions drawn are affected by methodological issues – were patients screened for depression, for example? What are the ethics of undertaking a prospective study with a patient, set alongside the impact of the death on relatives if undertaking a retrospective study? What is the effect of relying on staff accounts as to whether or not a patient has requested euthanasia or physician-assisted suicide? Nevertheless, the evidence appears to show that remarkably few requests are made for euthanasia by patients in palliative care (Kristjanson and Christakis, 2005). Of more recent interest is an exploration of the patient characteristics and experiences which lead, or might lead, to such requests. High levels of actual or anticipated pain, suffering and perceived diminished quality of life are associated with euthanasia requests or patients identifying that they might wish to have this option (Georges et al, 2005; Johansen et al, 2005). A small qualitative study in Hong Kong also identified high levels of existential distress as being associated with requests for euthanasia and suggested that such requests should not be taken at face value but the spiritual need addressed (Mak and Elwyn, 2005). One further point on which there is agreement is that patients' views appear to fluctuate and there is often ambivalence.

Attitudes of healthcare professionals

A recent survey generating 857 returns from doctors in the UK conducted by Clive Seale discovered that the popular belief that a lot of euthanasia is actually going on under the guise of end-of-life care technologies is actually not the case. The survey asked about voluntary euthanasia, physician-assisted suicide and ending life without an explicit request from the patient; low levels of all three practices were reported, with the UK having lower or similar rates compared with those reported in Belgium, Denmark, Italy, Holland, Sweden, Switzerland, Australia and New Zealand (Seale, 2006). This appears to reflect the attitudes reported in an earlier survey of British geriatricians, in which only 13 per cent said they would be willing to administer active voluntary euthanasia and only 12 per cent willing to provide physician-assisted suicide in some circumstances (Clark et al, 2001). A large survey of Swedish physicians employed in end-of-life settings reported that a third had administered drugs for pain and symptom control in doses likely to hasten death (Valverius et al, 2000).

Another large survey carried out in Hong Kong compared the views of the general public with those of doctors. Doctors were reported to agree in general with passive euthanasia (which they defined as withdrawing or withholding treatment), to be neutral about non-voluntary euthanasia (defined as when the patient cannot give consent through incapacity or coma), but opposed to active voluntary euthanasia. The general public, however, agreed with active voluntary euthanasia but disagreed with non-voluntary euthanasia and was neutral about passive euthanasia (Chong and Fok, 2005). The authors point out that lay persons are likely to be influenced by the Chinese culture which sees pain and suffering as being inflicted on the family as well as the individual, hence there may be a duty to remove this burden from one's relatives, whereas doctors are more likely to be influenced by their professional ethic and duty of care.

The attitudes of nurses have been separately studied. One of the reasons for this is that nurses have the closest day-to-day contact with patients and are involved in giving intimate care. Thus they are both the professional to whom patients and relatives may express their deep fears, anxieties and wishes, and also the one who may be there when they die, including as they 'slip away' under sedation. A nurse may well be the person to whom the patient voices a request for euthanasia (De Bal et al, 2005). One of the things that emerges in studies of nurses' attitudes to euthanasia and associated practices is the stress felt by many in the last stages of a patient's care. This may arise, for example, from feeling left to manage the implementation of decisions taken by others, from experiencing poor communication or differences of opinion with doctors, and from finding the care of a patient on terminal sedation an emotional burden with their therapeutic caring role removed (Morita et al, 2004). Demands for better training for all nurses in both ethics and palliative care (Doolan and Brown, 2004; Verpoort et al, 2004) relate to findings that working in palliative care significantly affects nurses' attitudes to euthanasia. Their greater expression of reservations, however, is significantly influenced by the success of palliative care in affording pain and symptom control (Verpoort et al, 2004). Even experienced palliative care nurses, opposed to euthanasia, are disturbed by the fact that some symptoms are still very difficult to control.

One US study of hospice nurses in Oregon found that once the question of physician-assisted suicide had been raised, the nurses felt increased responsibility to control symptoms completely, as though their ability to keep the patient comfortable was all that stood between them both and failure (Harvath et al, 2006). Some nurses felt that they had inadvertently been drawn into assisting patients with voluntary euthanasia – for example, by assisting them to control vomiting which then enabled them to take a lethal dose. Some nurses expressed regret that when euthanasia was chosen, it removed the opportunity for personal and family growth, spiritual transformation and reconciliation. This is a view clearly echoing the hospice philosophy of helping people to live until they die.

This Oregon study also, unusually, looked at the dilemmas experienced by social workers around euthanasia requests. Considering that social work has a long history of working with seriously ill and dying people, it is curious that the social work literature has largely ignored the issue of euthanasia and the impact that such requests might have on their relationships with dying and bereaved people (Arnold, 2004). The few empirical studies which have examined social workers' attitudes and practices around euthanasia (Ogden and Young, 1998 Csikai, 1999; Arnold, 2004) appear to show that social workers, when asked the direct question, largely reflect the predominant social attitude (for example, North Americans privileged the value of individual autonomy and the majority were in favour of legalising voluntary euthanasia and assisted suicide). But when asked to consider actual scenarios, or recount situations in which they had been involved, they demonstrate greater ambivalence (Leichtentritt, 2002; Arnold, 2004). This is unsurprising. Although they are not directly involved in the medical and physical aspects of care, social workers centre their engagement with dying people and their families on a psychosocial approach, which brings to the fore the effects of the illness and death on the dying person's life as a whole, most especially their relationships. They do this from a value base which prioritises the empowerment of the dying person. Thus it would seem likely that there would be some contradictions in these principles in practice around the question of euthanasia, not least because social work's family and social approach leads it to constantly seek to balance competing needs and rights.

A possible contradiction in the context of end-of-life care lies in social work's commitment to client self-determination and its sustaining role, which more recent articulations have seen as 'maintaining the spirit' (Lloyd, 2002) and palliative care social work has tended to see as the maintenance of hope. Arnold (2004) argues that further research is needed on the sources and meanings of hope in the context of life-threatening illness if social workers are to maintain this role in the current context of end-of-life care. Social work's commitment to anti-oppressive practice challenges the profession to engage with issues such as advance directives, treatment withdrawal or refusal and treatments to hasten death when performed on patients with diminished capacity or those who are incapable of giving consent. It is suggested that the profession must revise its various codes of ethics to take account of the contemporary treatment context (Mackelprang and Mackelprang, 2005). As with nurses, there are calls for training programmes to address these dilemmas, with the recognition that social workers are woefully ill-prepared for the issues which some service users may bring to the encounter in end-of-life care (Leichtentritt, 2002; Luptak, 2004).

A similar neglect is pointed to in the practice and training of rehabilitation professionals, who, it is argued, have no literature to assist them to grapple in practice with the dilemmas raised by euthanasia questions and genetic counselling programmes (Zanskas and Coduti, 2006). Rehabilitation professionals, such as speech, occupational and physiotherapists, work primarily outside of palliative care. They do, however, work with disabled people and people with long-term conditions of all ages and are at the centre of discussions about the potential for rehabilitation where there is a degenerative condition, or where the potential for recovery from an acute episode, such as a stroke, may be questioned. Both of these situations commonly occur in the frail older person who may be particularly vulnerable and disadvantaged. At the other end of the life cycle, rehabilitation has an important role to play in assisting parents with managing a child with multiple and complex impairments. Thus rehabilitation professionals are working in situations where legal and ethical dilemmas may frequently arise in decision making.

Conclusion

Twentieth-century developments in the care of people who are dying emerged out of deep concern about the attitudes and practices prevalent in the western world and entrenched in its hospitals, and the additional suffering which this caused to dying people and their families. Thus the hospice and palliative care movement has been underpinned by a valuing of the individual and philosophy of care which place their comfort and dignity at the centre. This led to a natural desire to define those characteristics which make for a 'good death'. However, that which grew out of the transforming influence of the hospice movement has been in danger of turning into the opposite – a restrictive template which pathologises those whose dying does not conform. In my own work I have referred to this as the 'tyranny' of the good death, appealing for a vision which embraces the 'good-enough-for-me' realities of most people (Lloyd, 1995). It is only as disquiet with reductionist versions of the good death has surfaced that scholarship has returned to the multifaceted roots of the concept. We are beginning to understand how 'dying well' for each individual requires a careful negotiation of these elements such that the dying is personally acceptable and the death has social meaning. Walters refers to this as 'dying with panache', including 'raging into the night' if this is how this person has lived their life and is their authentic death (Walters,

2004, p 408). But increasingly in our society the majority dying – the deaths of the very old – does not obviously have panache and does not fit with what Seale has termed the 'heroic' model of death (Seale, 1995b).

The importance of philosophical debate and the theoretical underpinnings for policy are just beginning to be recognised as crucial to the ongoing development of good end-of-life care and the ethical dilemmas contained therein. These confront practitioners on a daily basis, because one thing which *is* certain is that dying in the twenty-first century is for the most part a managed process. This is one reason why deaths which occur outside of that process are so difficult to accommodate within our ontological frame. Policy in health and social care is notoriously under-theorised and our neglect of the philosophical dimension has been at the expense of considerable ethical discomfort experienced by those people charged with implementing policy and providing hands-on care. When this is end-of-life care, it touches the deepest personal concerns and instincts and is governed by cultural imperatives. Yet although the importance of religious ethic, philosophical standpoint and cultural context are acknowledged and represented in the debates about end-of-life care, technologies and euthanasia, the empirical research is still relatively sparse on the significance of religion, beliefs and culture on the wishes and choices which dying people and their relatives express, or professionals promote.

This chapter has also shown how services for people who are dying are shaped by the overall climate of health and social care. In summary, the key thrusts are:

- to enable people to receive palliative care while remaining at home for as long as they choose, including to die at home if possible;
- to extend the remit of palliative care to non-cancers including the diseases of old age;
- to facilitate individual choice and the full involvement of the dying person and their family in treatment decisions;
- to reach out to minority groups and make mainstream services culturally appropriate;
- to further define and demonstrate in practice the outworkings of the principles of holistic care;
- to make hospices a fully integrated part of the health and social care network.

Some elements and positions in the issues we have discussed are irreconcilable. It is the task of the legislators and policy makers to negotiate a path which is acceptable to the majority and allows minority viewpoints to be respected wherever and as far as is possible. Ultimately, the arguments put forward against the Joffe Bill in the UK in its first incarnation were a mixture of moral, religious and pragmatic (Neuberger, 2006). However, legislation and policy may determine the framework which governs care of the dying, but patients and service users and health and social care practitioners alike contribute their experience and expertise to the environment in which that dying takes place. There remains an acute shortage of specialist palliative care practitioners across the world and this must be addressed. There is also, however, continuing evidence that too many health and social care professionals outside of palliative care are ignorant of the philosophy and practice which constitutes sensitive, culturally competent and quality care for people nearing the end of life. Only so equipped can professionals in all sectors of health and social care negotiate the complex choices and issues involved in contemporary dying – for themselves as well as for those they seek to help.

Key questions for practitioners

1. What have you learnt from this chapter about approaches to the care of people who are dying and how might this affect your work?
2. Do you come across any of the ethical dilemmas discussed here and how do you currently resolve them?
3. Is there anything in the positions discussed here which might help you deal better with your dilemma(s)?
4. Does end-of-life care planning feature in your direct work with service users? If not, why not? Should it?
5. How well does the service in which you work address the needs of people from ethnic minorities?
6. How well does it address spiritual and religious needs?
7. What further knowledge/skills do you need to gain in order to improve your practice with people at the end of life and their families?

Note

[1] But see Chapter Two for discussion of the reduction in 'terminal' diagnoses due to progress in treating malignant conditions.

SIX

Dying and bereavement in old age

Introduction

At first sight, dying in old age presents the most timely and natural of all deaths and the accompanying bereavement the most anticipated and uncomplicated grief. Perhaps for this reason, there has historically been a notable neglect of the topic. Research into ageing, despite its mushrooming in the latter part of the twentieth century, largely ignored the subject of death until it became apparent that the health and social care of older people might merge seamlessly into end-of-life care. The seminal work on dying and grief which we looked at earlier was either based on younger populations, such as younger cancer sufferers or those bereaved through public disaster, or the inclusion of large numbers of older people, such as older widows, was coincidental and the lens of old age did not provide an explicit angle in the theorising. The counselling textbooks continue to pay little attention to the dimension of old age, although, by comparison, new resources for working with children and young people in grief appear all the time. Yet for most of us in the advanced societies of late modernity, our first and only encounters with death will occur in conjunction with old age, as we experience the deaths of grandparents, aged parents, partners, siblings and friends who have reached old age, to finally face our own death. The majority of people in the Anglo-Saxon and North American worlds currently die aged 75 or above and the proportions dying at over 85 years are set to rise. Death is in one sense ever-present for those working with older people, yet at the same time invisible in older people's services.

Moreover, it is becoming increasingly apparent that what at first sight appears simply the natural order of things is often a complex, difficult process, both for those older people and their relatives who are dying or bereaved, and for the professional carers and services that seek to assist in managing the end of a long life. One of the problems for the current 'oldest old' is that there has been little opportunity to observe this phase in previous generations. Thus, they may come to their own dying unprepared, already beyond the point when they can 'set their affairs in order' – practically, emotionally, psychologically and spiritually – at least on their own initiative. The transition into the end of life and the care which it requires may be rather less of a seamless join and rather more of an uncomfortable jolt. The sociolegal-ethical issues are complicated by the vulnerability induced by frailty and common conditions of old age such as dementia. The fact that people are living longer, but with increasing frailty and health problems, has produced a cohort of the 'oldest old' for which we are socially unprepared at the same time as an emphasis on getting the maximum out of life in old age seems to inhibit active engagement with the business of dying. When these old people die, their removal from our emotional, psychological and social space where they have been an assumed presence for so long often causes a disruption for which the bereaved are ill-prepared. For those who remain but are themselves old, the material and social resources for carrying on can seem impossibly limited. For all these reasons, it is vital that we develop a more sophisticated understanding of death in old age. That understanding must take account of the fact that neither living nor dying in old age are completely homogeneous experiences. They are crucially mediated by gender, ethnicity, socioeconomic variables, health status and cultural and religious factors.

Death in old age in the UK

In England and Wales, of 512,541 deaths in 2004, 169,793 or 33 per cent were of people aged 75–84 and 153,879 or 30 per cent of those aged over 85 (Mortality Statistics Series DH1 no 37, ONS 2006). As shown by Table 6.1, however, there are differences between the sexes with far more women living longer and dying at age 85 and over.

Table 6.1: Elderly deaths 2004, by gender

	Numbers			Percentages	
	All ages	Age 75–84	Age 85 and over	Age 75–84	Age 85 and over
Male	244,130	87,266	51,239	35.8	21.0
Female	268,411	82,537	102,640	30.8	38.2
Total	512,541	169,793	153,879	33.1	30.0

Source: Mortality Statistics Series DH1 no 37, ONS 2006

The main cause of death among the elderly for both men and women and in both age groups is circulatory problems, as shown in Figure 6.1. Respiratory diseases are a lesser cause and diseases of the digestive system relatively unimportant across age and gender. Cancer is a major cause for males aged 75–84 but relatively unimportant for females aged 85 and over. Other causes are more important in the older age group, particularly for women. The most important of these other causes are mental and behavioural disorders and symptoms not otherwise classified, particularly for women, and diseases of the genito-urinary system, which are slightly more significant for men.

Although deaths among elderly people from all causes as a proportion of all deaths vary with gender and age group, the proportions also vary with different causes of death. Figure 6.2 shows that circulatory and respiratory diseases among females aged 75–84 account for over one third of deaths at all ages from these causes, but at age 85 and over this rises to nearly half. Cancers and digestive

Figure 6.1: Causes of death 2004, by age group and gender

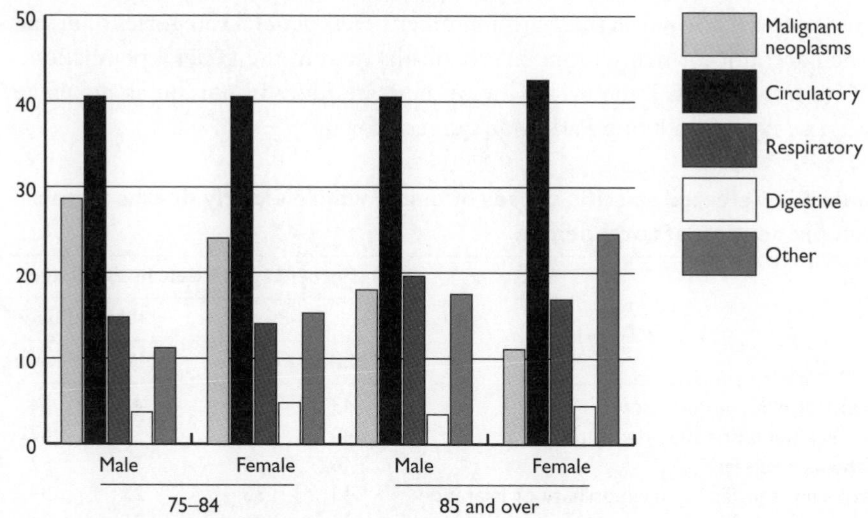

Source: Mortality Statistics Series DH1 no 37, ONS 2006

Figure 6.2: Causes of death in the elderly in relation to deaths at all ages

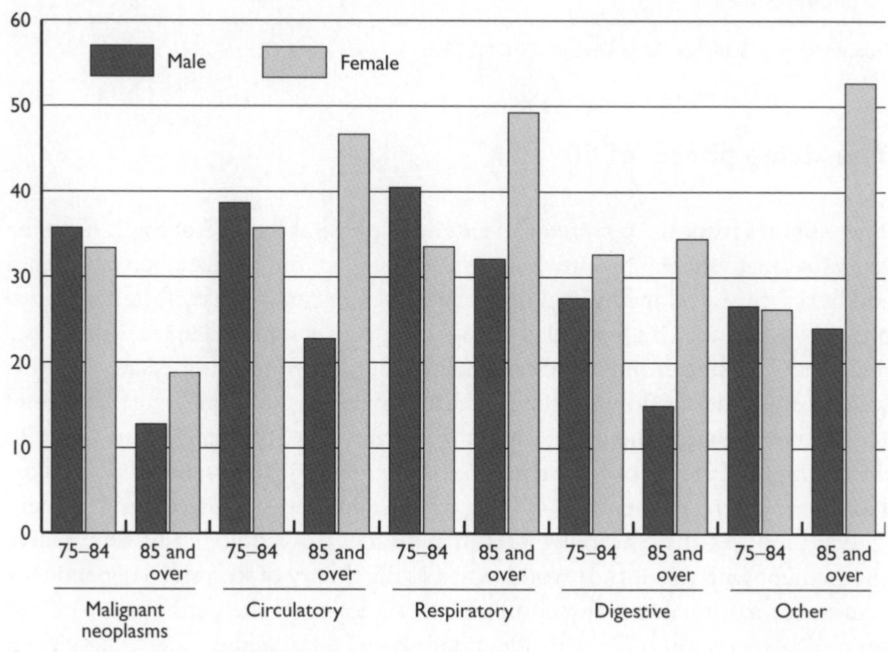

Source: Mortality Statistics Series DH1 no 37, ONS 2006

diseases of males aged 85 and over on the other hand are the cause of death for only about one sixth of all deaths from these disorders.

Although numbers are small and the proportions of deaths within the elderly age groups are also small, there are a number of less general categories of diseases which account for many more elderly deaths than in the general population. A selection is listed in Table 6.2. Many of these are more important at age 85 and over, the exception being Parkinson's disease for men.

Table 6.2: Selected specific causes of death where elderly deaths form high proportion of total deaths

	Percentage of deaths at all ages			
	75–84		85 and over	
	Male	Female	Male	Female
Intestinal infectious diseases	43	35	41	54
Vascular and unspecified dementia	40	29	50	67
Alzheimer's disease	46	39	36	52
Stroke not specified as haemorrhage or infarction	45	36	33	54
Other heart diseases	35	31	31	54
Atherosclerosis	38	24	41	71
Pneumonia	36	27	45	64
Osteoporosis	30	28	58	67
Renal failure	39	34	36	50
Senility	16	10	83	90
Falls	31	32	22	45
Parkinson's disease	53	45	28	45

Source: Mortality Statistics Series DH1 no 37, ONS 2006

The 'dying phase' of life

These figures paint the picture of an extended phase at the end of life. It has been suggested that whereas primitive societies created a liminal phase between death and burial, the developed world in the twenty-first century has created a liminal phase *before* death. This 'extended dying' creates issues and dilemmas for us as a society and for health and social care practitioners. The most immediate dilemma we encounter has to do with the fact that the emphasis on quality of life in old age has not included the idea of moving towards death. In part, this is down to the triumph of the theory of 'structured dependency' (Townsend, 1981; Walker, 1981) over 'disengagement theory' (Cumming and Henry, 1961). Disengagement theory proposes that the older person withdraws psychologically from active engagement with the outside world, whereas the theory of structured dependency argues that marginality is forced upon older people by the construction of old age as a socioeconomically dependent state. Most social gerontologists have been opposed to the idea originally proposed by Midwinter that there are 'layers' of ageing represented by the 'young old', the 'old' and the 'oldest old' (Midwinter, 1987). However, the situation in which we now find ourselves, with life prolonged for increasing numbers of people but with higher levels of disability and with both chronic and acute health problems, should lead us to reconsider too monolithic an approach to this final phase of life.

Attitudes to death

Repeated psychological studies have shown that, in general, people are more likely to think about death the older they get. This is perhaps unsurprising, although it does run counter to current assertions that older people are more concerned with quality of life than anticipating death. If we consider the different strands identified in Chapter Three – *awareness of death, meanings attributed to death, fear of death* and *preparation for death* – the relatively limited research which focuses specifically on older people continues to find that they are more likely to consider their own death and to make preparation for it than younger people.

In her ethnographic study undertaken in care homes in the north-east of England, Hockey records many instances of residents making reference to their own death, ranging from the savage – requests to be 'finished off' – to the matter-of-fact – 'it's to be expected any time at my age' – to the jest – mimicking death for the benefit of care attendants (Hockey and James, 1993). Other studies have shown that the 'oldest old' group, in particular, do contemplate and accept the inevitability of their own death (Johnson and Barer, 1997; Field, 2000; Cicirelli, 2001). Nevertheless, Williams' study of older Aberdonians (in Scotland) emphasises that this is not a generation passively awaiting their deaths.

The meanings attributed to death and fear of death show remarkable consistency over age. Older people's views about what makes for a 'good' or a 'bad' death are not particularly different from the thinking of younger cohorts, and there is also remarkable consistency across cultures on some core features that they wish for (such as to be surrounded by family and at peace), and things they want to avoid (such as a painful and undignified death) (Holloway et al, 2005). Two points distinguish older people's attitudes, however. First, older people are especially conscious of not wanting to be a burden on family. This was a surprising finding of a study of older Chinese people in the UK, where the tradition of 'filial piety' appeared to have been reversed (Chapman et al, 2005). Second, where fear of death is expressed, it shifts from the existential issue of 'non-being' found among younger people, to fear of dying (although existential fears remain for those believing death to represent extinction; Cicirelli, 2001). Differences arising from gender or ethnic group also relate to dying itself, one possible interpretation being that they reflect the realities of end-of-life care for these groups (Depaola et al, 2003). Thus an acceptance of death itself still leaves open a wide range of concerns about the dying process (Howarth, 1998). Williams (1990) found some contradictions in thinking on the good or bad death; for example, whilst it was good to 'go quickly', knowing little about the process, it was also good to have one's family around and to have made proper preparation for death. Contradictory attitudes were particularly evident when it came to views on technologies to hasten death.

Religion and spirituality

One area in which older people's attitudes are thought to be distinguished is their religiosity and spiritual awareness. There is a growing interest in the 'spirituality of ageing' (Jewell, 1999; MacKinlay, 2001) and we cannot do justice to it here. However, there is not much which focuses specifically on the overlap with death – although in some senses it is all about death in that the underlying assumption is that approaching death heightens older people's awareness of their spiritual selves and personal belief systems. The spirituality of ageing explores themes which recur in this book, such as personhood, continuity (of relationships and identities), sense of self, meaning-making, personal growth and fostering inner resources. What should not be assumed is that these necessarily imply a religious or spiritual life for the individual older person.

Equally, religion should not be dismissed as barely relevant for most older people in our secularised society. Rather, the declining role of religion and the church in western Christendom may have removed for many older people the moral, philosophical and social underpinnings which traditionally structured and sustained their experience of death. There is evidence that older people struggle without this framework, even when they personally had found the traditional beliefs to be unsatisfactory and had rejected the involvement of the church in their lives (Williams, 1990; Coleman et al, 2004). Some show a return to beliefs handed down in childhood when faced with a terminal diagnosis or bereavement (Lloyd, 1996). The loss of a wider existential framework within which to locate their experiences of dying and bereavement may well be significant for older people, but it has been given little attention in either the theorising of dying and bereavement or the development of practice interventions. Considerable attention *has* been paid to specific religion-related variables in the US research. Lund (1989b) concludes that they do not of themselves explain the diversity of responses to bereavement observed in older people. One final, but important, point should always be borne in mind by health and social care practitioners in contact with older people around the time of a death. For many older people from non-western and southern European cultures, religion is a way of life and belief in life after death requires that they should make preparation for death (Firth, 1999).

Suicide

A rarely reported fact is that contemplation of their life and their future leads some older people to contemplate their death and commit suicide. Double suicides, involving both partners in a suicide pact, are reported to occur most frequently amongst older people (Salvatore, 1999–2001). Suicides of older people are said to account for disproportionately high numbers of all suicides in Britain, Australia and the US (Samaritans, 1990; Kissane and McLaren, 2006). What little we know about this phenomenon suggests that it is associated with depression, sometimes alcoholism, and existential issues such as feeling cut off from the rest of society, feeling useless, helpless, and not valued by their families. There is no evidence to suggest that having a terminal illness is a predictor of suicide and, in fact, some suggestion that older people are more accepting of a terminal diagnosis (Young and Cullen, 1996) and less in favour of euthanasia (Catt et al, 2005) than younger people. That suicidal feelings arise from the circumstances of being old in youth-oriented cultures might be reasonably surmised. The problem with which we started this chapter, that medical advances have created a liminal phase for the old without the social apparatus or know-how to manage it, may also lie behind this disturbing problem.

Care at the end of life

There is an increasing body of work about end-of-life care (as distinct from palliative care) which deals more broadly with a range of social and healthcare issues and is based on older populations. Far from representing an offshoot set of concerns, end-of-life care for older people crystallises the central dilemmas in contemporary dying.

Place of death

The statistics on place of death provide a snapshot picture of what is currently happening in policy and practice regarding services for older people at the end of life. The most frequent place of death for men and women of both older age groups in the UK is 'Other hospitals'. For those aged 75–84 the second most frequent place of death is at home. However, for females aged 85 and over 'Other' places are more important, mainly other communal establishments. Hospices feature more for males aged 85 and over than for other genders or age groups.

Drawing on figures from the Office of National Statistics for Wales, Ahmad and O'Mahoney (2005) point to a shift from dying at home to dying in care homes or hospital, identifying that over the twenty-year period from 1981 to 2001, both the numbers and percentage of deaths of older people occurring in the community fell steadily, while the percentages of deaths in hospital and care homes both rose. These trends were more marked for those over the age of 85. Interestingly, care home deaths peaked in the mid-1980s, whereas hospital deaths have continued to rise, particularly for the oldest group. This pattern is reflected outside of the UK. Various studies across the US, Australia and Europe found a similar shift from home to institution in older people's dying, and further identified that the oldest old, women and single people are less likely to die at home (Grande et al, 1998; Steele et al, 1999; Klinkenberg et al, 2005).

Figure 6.3: Places of death, by age group

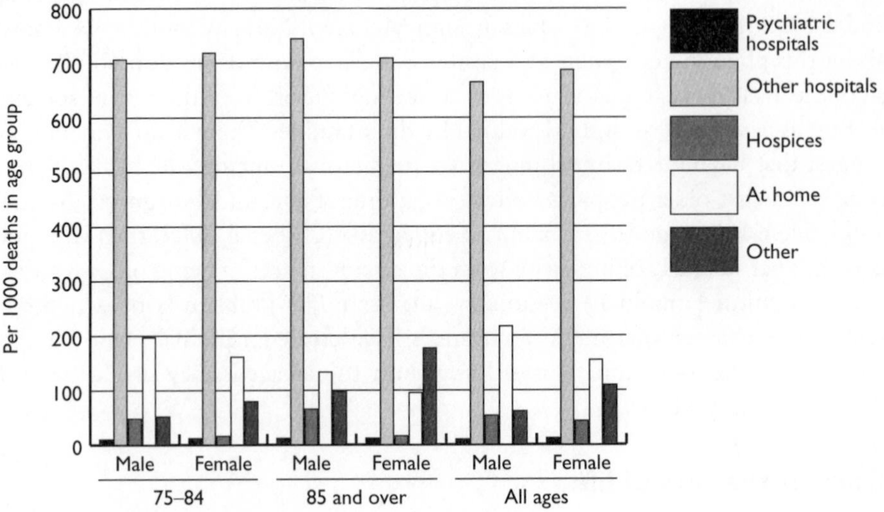

Source: Mortality Statistics Series DH1 no 37, ONS 2006

Thus the concentration of death in the oldest old in the western world means that we are increasingly looking at older people dying in residential or nursing home care, or hospital. As with hospices, however, it is common for the older person to be admitted to hospital only in the last weeks or even days of life. In their population-based study (that is, not confined to those with a terminal diagnosis or in receipt of palliative care), undertaken as part of the Longitudinal Ageing Study Amsterdam, Klinkenberg et al (2005) noted that 37 per cent of the older people were living in institutional care at the time of their death, but this figure rose to half of the sample of the oldest old (those with a mean age of 85 years). Moreover, around half were moved from one care setting to another in the last three months of their life. Most commonly, this was hospitalisation for people previously living at home or in residential care, or into nursing home care from hospital. The authors hypothesise that having a limited social network increases the risk of hospital admission occurring in the last week of life. A study of admissions to a hospital in New South Wales, Australia, found that most older patients had multiple admissions in the last year of their life (Chan et al, 2003), and an American study (Steele et al, 1999) estimated that a third of Americans will 'pass through' a long-term care facility before they die. Thus, not only are older people ending their days in an institutional setting, their last months and weeks are frequently characterised by considerable instability.

One final piece of information is crucial. Figures for palliative care service users in the UK show that older people are disproportionately under-represented, even when this is looked at in terms of cancer sufferers alone (Higginson et al, 1998; Catt et al, 2005). This is especially marked in the over 85s, who constituted

15 per cent of all cancer deaths in 2000/01, but only 9 per cent were cared for by hospice or specialist palliative care services. Thus, in so far as specialist care can be determined from the setting in which they die, older people appear to be considerably disadvantaged.

Older people's preferences for place of death

Exploring older people's expressed preferences concerning place of death gives us some idea of the sort of care they would want to have. Studies in both the UK and the US suggest that most people would prefer to die at home (Townsend et al, 1990; Fried et al, 1999). However, the picture is rather more nuanced when these responses are probed, and a small amount of more recent research indicates that older people's choices are dependent upon a number of situational factors, and that their choices may change with worsening disease and disability. Martineau et al (2003) summarise the most commonly cited factors affecting choices as being the availability of family support and professional help, the functional condition of the older person and the prognosis for any concomitant disease.

One of the problems in gauging older people's views is that it is extremely difficult to collect data from older people who are at the point of needing end-of-life care. Thus to a large extent the views expressed arise from older people's observations of someone else's dying, often when they themselves were in the role of carer or closest relative. This inevitably lends a certain twist to their opinions. In a study which recruited a representative sample of people over the age of 55 from GP practices in London, but excluded any who were seriously ill, researchers found a slight preference for hospice care over dying at home or in hospital, but also found that those over the age of 75 preferred to die in hospital rather than at home, whereas the younger group preferred home to hospital (Catt et al, 2005). A contemporaneous study, also with older people who were not actually receiving palliative care services, undertaken in a northern England city reported that older people chose home as their preferred place of death, but only in ideal circumstances. They expressed reservations about being too much of a burden on family and friends, particularly if these became involved in delivering a high degree of personal and even nursing care. Equally, a number of people were uncomfortable with the idea of too much professional and 'high-tech' care being provided in the home because then it would no longer feel like home. The researchers on this study went on to identify what 'home' actually meant. It seemed that the notion of dying at home comprised a number of features – such as having one's loved ones around and enjoying flexible routines – rather than being fixed to the geographical space (Gott et al, 2004).

Thus it appears that many older people are dubious about dying at home if the care is not adequate or places too much of a burden on relatives. Examining and comparing ways in which death is handled in particular care settings sheds further light on the dying experiences of older people.

Dying in residential or nursing homes

In a participant observation study in an elderly care home in the north of England undertaken in the 1980s, Jenny Hockey identified that although the residents themselves made reference to their own (impending) deaths, staff dealt with the issue by applying the labels 'fit' or 'frail' (Hockey, 1990). Once an individual had passed into the 'frail' category, they were treated as no longer needing to participate in the ongoing life of the home, consigned to that limbo state which others have categorised as 'social death'. Some ten years later, a study undertaken in English nursing homes in which staff had received specific training in palliative care reached very similar conclusions about the strategies used by staff to manage the transition from living to dying (Froggatt, 2001). Staff were observed to use the term 'poorly' to refer to someone who was thought to be dying, perhaps following a critical event such as a stroke. However, perhaps because of advances in medical care and its greater availability in nursing homes than when Hockey undertook her study, there appeared to be greater uncertainty about the actual timing of death with many residents lingering for a long time in the 'poorly' category whilst others were restored to the active category. Thus, creating and managing the transitional state was all-important to staff. This is marginally different from the creation of a 'dying space' which Hockey had observed, but what both studies demonstrate is the need of staff to control dying when it occurs in a confined and controlled space (physical and social) alongside the living.

For the older person, such treatment might very well seem like a denial of their death, at the same time as they are deemed to have passed beyond living. This is somewhat surprising, given that staff in this study had received the training in palliative care which is recommended to equip care staff in nursing and residential homes to provide sensitive end-of-life care (Sidell et al, 1997) and that death in old age when faculties and functions are failing is seen by most care staff to be both timely and natural (Komaromy and Hockey, 2001). Another recent study provides further evidence of the ways in which staff in residential and nursing homes simultaneously deny death as they seek to manage it. Residents were observed to be fully aware that a death had occurred, because they overheard conversations or the sounds of the corpse being removed, but elaborate measures were taken to ensure that no one saw the dead body, or, indeed, anything which might point to a death (Komaromy, 2000). A recent Swedish study links the lack of openness about dying in nursing homes to an undermining of the dignity of the residents (Franklin et al, 2006). The authors of this Swedish study conclude that older people's fears about their changing body as they become increasingly frail and physically dependent, escalate as they approach death and threaten their sense of inner self.

Dying in hospital

What of the hospital as a place for older people to die? Given the likelihood of an older person, particularly the 'oldest old', spending at least the last few days of their life in hospital, it is important that we consider what this might mean. Unfortunately, there is very little research to inform our understanding of death in hospital as it currently occurs, perhaps as a consequence of the high profile of the hospice movement, representing the ideal 'good' dying, where hospitals had seemed to epitomise all that was bad about modern dying. Thus we are in danger of ignoring the reality for most people of dying in hospital. Costello suggests that there is huge variation in the end-of-life care afforded to older people dying in hospital and we are still unclear about what constitutes a 'good death' in hospital with nurses having little to guide their practice (Costello, 2006). There seems to be rather more consensus around what constitutes a 'bad death', marked by a lack of dignity and out-of-control symptoms. In fact, most of the literature is concerned to construct the polarised types of 'good' and 'bad' death as experienced by nursing and other front-line staff. As we explored in Chapter Three, nurses feel the experience has been good if the nurses have been able to prepare themselves and the family properly, infuse the death with individual meaning, and it occurs as a managed social event on the ward (Low and Payne, 1996; McNamara, 2001; Hopkinson et al, 2005). However, Costello's study of the care of older patients in specialist elderly care hospital settings found that care of those who were dying was characterised by a lack of meaningful communication with the individual older person; a tendency to see 'quality time' and quality care in terms of time spent attending to physical needs, leading to consternation when the patient died during a busy or handover period on the ward; and inhibited relationships with families arising from the need to defer to the opinion of doctors about what should or should not be said, by whom and when (Costello, 2001 and 2006).

It appears that older patients, although cared for on wards specifically set up to provide integrated old-age medicine and thus in accordance with 'best practice' principles, may not be getting that holistic care in their dying which is regarded as best practice in palliative care. Further, the nurses caring for them may be frustrated by organisational and resource constraints (Taylor, 2001). One further point should be emphasised here. At the heart of the notion of the good death is the control of pain – and this is a notion which seems to have cross-cultural currency (Seymour et al, forthcoming). One of the concerns expressed by older people about dying at home is that pain may not be adequately controlled (Gott et al, 2004). A Canadian study found that 69 per cent of respondents favoured hospital care when faced with pain (Martineau et al, 2003). Yet serious doubts have been raised, internationally, about the extent to which older people, particularly those dying from conditions other than cancer, have their pain adequately controlled (Lynn et al, 1997; Addington-Hall and Altman, 2000; Davies and Higginson, 2004; Seymour et al, 2007). There is evidence that when the older person has dementia, or is otherwise impaired in their ability to convey their experience, the assessment and treatment of their pain is even more neglected (Fox et al, 1999).

Whilst this picture of dying in hospital has drawn on studies conducted on older people's wards, it should be remembered that most older people arrive at hospital, for what turns out to be the last time, as an 'emergency' admission after some critical health event. In such circumstances they will usually be found a bed wherever one is available, and only moved on to the appropriate specialist ward as and when a bed becomes free. Given the average short final stays of these older patients, many will not be moved and will die on these general wards. We do not as yet know enough about their actual dying experience. Death in hospital as the final stage of care when one is old is the majority pattern of dying at present, in advanced societies, and likely to be the overwhelming pattern for the future, quite probably in general healthcare settings. It is imperative that contemporary palliative care expands its vision to encompass this context for dying in old age.

Palliative care

Although older people have relatively little access to specialist palliative care services at present, there are moves to transfer the principles and practice of palliative care into recognised older people's care settings, such as stroke care. Stroke is the third commonest cause of death in developed countries and around 30 per cent of stroke patients in the UK die in the first month and most in the first 10 days (figures quoted in Jack et al, 2004). A small study piloted the use of the Liverpool dying pathway (described in Chapter Five) on a stroke unit. In several key areas of care, improvements were shown when the pathway was implemented – for example, in discontinuing inappropriate interventions and medication, keeping relatives informed as death approached. One of the continuing hindrances in this approach is in identifying older people who are dying and would benefit from palliative care but who are suffering from non-malignant disease (Addington-Hall, 1998). Refusal, or inability, to acknowledge that such people are in the 'dying phase' is part and parcel of the denial of death which we observed in nursing home culture. This has a number of negative and discriminatory consequences for older people, not least in relation to the control of pain. The London study referred to earlier (Catt et al, 2005) reported that across all age groups, these older people wanted pain relief even if it left them confused. The growing evidence that older people are discriminated against in terms of good palliative care and specifically, in not receiving adequate pain relief, is particularly disturbing in the light of these and similar findings.

Technological and managed death

It is in the end-of-life care of older people that the questions raised by medical advances, which make it possible to prolong life, and the decisions and choices about what care should be provided, are routinely faced. Chapter Five explored these questions in their broad philosophical, social, legal and ethical contexts. There are three angles which are particularly relevant to older people:

- When should active treatment aimed at 'cure' cease, and who should make that decision?
- Should steps be taken to hasten death, and who should make that decision?
- How should older people be consulted about their care and what is the 'currency' of previously expressed wishes?

Central to these questions is the quality of life of the older person as they progress through the dying phase of life.

Perhaps the starting point in this enormously complicated area is the extent to which doctors pursue treatment, including so-called 'aggressive' treatments, with older people, and the extent to which older people wish them to do so, including when they are seriously ill with a terminal diagnosis. Underlying this is the question of whether or not the diagnosis and prognosis is shared, and with whom. Costello (2006) found that even in these days of supposed open communication between doctors and patients, it was common for relatives to be told but not the older person, and, often, for there to be no open communication at all but rather everyone working to a set of assumptions that the older person is dying. An American study which compared the treatment of older patients with dementia with a group that had cancer, looked at a range of 'aggressive' life-prolonging interventions, including cardiopulmonary resuscitation, systemic antiobiotics and do not resuscitate orders. The study found that, overall, 47 per cent were given 'invasive non-palliative' treatments and that cardiopulmonary resuscitation was given out of all proportion to expected survival (Ahronheim et al, 1996). A more recent study in New South Wales, Australia, looked at the combination of care plans and not for resuscitation (NFR)[1] orders in the last year of life of 110 patients with an average age of 80 (Chan et al, 2003). Sixty-one of these patients had both a care plan and NFR order, 91 per cent having been written just prior to their death; 88 had one or other documented. These plans were most frequently associated with diagnoses of cardiac failure, cancer and dementia, with strokes and fractures also featuring strongly in the histories. However, only eight patients had an 'advanced care plan', that is, a care plan documented *prior* to their last hospital stay.

This picture should cause us to reflect. The authors infer that, given that advanced care plans are clinician-driven, there is no certainty that they had been discussed with the patient, especially given the stage at which most of the care plans were documented. They cite other studies which show that care plans and NFR orders are rarely discussed until the last hospital admission and that patient and family treatment preferences are then poorly documented. Given that the majority of older people in the western world are admitted to hospital a few days or weeks before their death, frequently after a stroke or fall, and that cardiac failure, certain forms of cancer and dementia are the common diseases and disorders of old age, we can conjecture that this picture of clinician-driven care plans, introduced at a stage when discussion with the older person may be difficult or impossible, is potentially widespread practice. Certainly it should lead us to look very carefully at how older people can be meaningfully involved in decisions about their end-of-life care. Particular ethical and practical issues are presented when the older person also has dementia.

The most common dilemmas raised for the medical practitioner in particular concern the questions of physician-assisted death (PAD) and whether or not to provide, or when to withdraw, artificial nutrition and hydration (ANH) – tube feeding, in layperson's speak. In addition to the fundamental issues posed for doctors of hastening death rather than preserving life, geriatricians display particular caution about both these practices. Physician-assisted death as it relates to older people is most likely brought about by practices such as prescribing current medication at such a level as to likely hasten death (referred to as double effect in the report of the House of Lords Select Committee on Medical Ethics, 1993-94). A survey of the views of consultant geriatricians undertaken through the membership of the British Geriatrics Society in 1999 showed 68 per cent to be opposed to PAD on ethical grounds, only 12 per cent saying that they would be willing to provide such assistance in some cases (Clark et al, 2001). The authors of this study quote evidence from the US, Canada and Italy which demonstrates similar reluctance amongst physicians to engage in PAD, although these studies were not specific to the older population. Additional comments in the UK study indicated a strong preference for promoting good palliative care for older people, and an inclination to deal with these issues on a case-by-case basis as part of the doctor–patient (and family) relationship. There was in all the studies quoted a desire for legislative controls, however, and, in the UK study, this was specifically linked to concerns about abuses of the practice where vulnerable older people are involved. Eighty-four per cent felt that if the practice of PAD and also active voluntary euthanasia (AVE) were legal, many older people would be pressurised into this course of action by their families.

This discussion assumes that the older person is involved in making a request to be helped to die. Those receiving artificial nutrition and hydration are usually not in a position to express a view about their continuing care. The American literature has been particularly concerned with ANH, where it is claimed that aggressive tube-feeding treatments are pursued as the norm for patients with severe dementia (Ahronheim et al, 1996; Hoefler, 2000), with decisions about tube feeding often made late in the day and in haste. Hoefler (2000) suggests that nasogastric tubes (which are preferred for a number of clinical reasons to stomach tubes) are often frightening for the patient with dementia, and their consequent behaviour in trying to remove the tube results in restraint mechanisms being used. Hoefler concludes that artificial feeding is a problematic procedure in itself and merely adds to the distress of the dying patient. This conclusion is supported by others, including an American team of researchers who have investigated a number of angles associated with ANH and conclude that, in any case, tube feeding does not appear to be the factor prolonging survival (Sieger et al, 2002). Perhaps most disturbingly, this article reports findings showing that patients with severe dementia are more likely to be treated with feeding tubes than those who have the capacity to discuss treatment options, and suggests that the way in which legislation is constructed, and the litigious context of US healthcare, militates against physicians offering best palliative care for older people who lack decision-making capacity. Moreover, it has been suggested (Huang and Ahronheim, 2000) that many healthcare professionals are unclear about both the clinical practice and underpinning principles of artificial nutrition and hydration.

In the UK, the more contentious issues have been around older people being 'allowed' to die through neglect by their carers. A long-running high-profile case in the UK about the nursing care of patients with dementia eventually concluded that nurses had not been negligent in failing to see to the nutrition needs of these older patients. However, the case provoked considerable public debate about it being common practice for very old and/or confused patients to be 'allowed to die' simply because they cannot attend to their own feeding and insufficient time and attention is available from nursing and care home staff to ensure that their nutritional needs are being met.

In order to be able to influence their care when they are no longer able to participate actively in making decisions, some (older) people draw up living wills, otherwise known as advance directives. Others may make advance statements expressing their wishes and views on particular treatments, although the latter are generally not legally binding in the way in which an advance directive is. Most commonly, these deal with issues such as the circumstances in which they might wish to be given life-prolonging treatments and when they would wish these to cease, the circumstances in which they would or would not wish to be resuscitated, particular treatments which they would or would not find acceptable, and identifying of any particular beliefs affecting or dictating their end-of-life care and management of their death. A study conducted in a London hospital with 74 older patients (Schiff et al, 2000) found that most older people lacked knowledge about such possibilities, but 74 per cent expressed an interest in writing a living will when this option was explained to them. People liked the idea of ensuring that their views were known and thought having a living will would relieve their family of the burden of decision making (although the majority also chose a relative as their healthcare proxy, in the event of one being needed). Age Concern England has responded to a growing interest in advance directives and statements by producing a fact sheet (Age Concern, 2005).

The relatively small number of UK studies in this area have been concerned to discover older people's preferences more broadly concerning their end-of-life care. As already noted, the control of pain is a central concern that is repeatedly stated. The Sheffield study referred to earlier in this chapter provides accounts of older people (or their relatives) struggling to get hospital staff to prescribe or administer medication to control their pain, which they believed to be available but being withheld. In this connection, participants displayed some confusion about whether adequate pain relief belonged to basic palliative care, or tipped over into a deliberate 'hastening' of death. The oldest old group in the London General Practice study (Catt et al, 2005) tended to oppose physician-assisted suicide although the younger group did not. However, the overwhelming majority of persons in the study which asked about living wills (Schiff et al, 2000) said that they would refuse surgery, artificial feeding and hydration, ventilation, resuscitation and antibiotics, if and when they reached the end stage of a terminal disease.

There is much more data available about the preferences of older Americans (for example, Gamble et al, 1991; Elder et al, 1992). However, more recent US work alerts us to the mistake of assuming that such attitudes have enduring currency and that they are generalisable. Preferences expressed have been shown to be heavily context-dependent in terms of social and philosophical climate, individual psychosocial characteristics and ethnic/community grouping. So, for example, older Americans generally appear to be moving slowly towards favouring the legalisation of voluntary euthanasia and assisted suicide, but Cicirelli and MacLean (2000) found views on extending life, refusing treatment and assisted suicide among terminally ill older people in Indiana to be significantly influenced by religiosity, valuing of the preservation of life, valuing of quality of life, fear of death and views about the locus of control. Another study, undertaken among older people living in the community in Arizona, suggested that in addition to health and social contextual factors, personal development factors also influenced end-of-life preferences. A category which the authors describe as 'integrated moral reasoning' also emerged as significant (Decker and Reed, 2005). This suggests a growing level of social awareness and public debate about end-of-life decisions, which is likely to produce continuing shifts in opinion.

The palliative care movement has generally opposed advance directives, particularly where this incorporates requests for voluntary euthanasia and assisted suicide. The argument is put forward that people do not know how they will feel until actually in that situation, and much may depend on the quality of care which they receive, and hence their quality of dying. Equally, it should be remembered that emotional and physical distress, experienced by either or both the dying person and their family in the last stages of life, may significantly influence the decisions made. The Sheffield study found participants cautious about whether or not they would want to hold to an advance directive when they reached that point (Seymour, 2003). The possibility of people changing their minds, and what factors might influence them to do so, is an important issue. Already, when individuals' views on specific treatments are taken over intervals of up to two years, they have been found to be only moderately stable (quoted in Lockhart et al, 2001). Longer periods of time in which both the treatments and the context of care may change quite markedly pose a quite different scenario in terms of adherence to advance directives, particularly since the likelihood is that advances in medical treatments may elongate still further the period of gradual decline in old age. At what point should the expression of a view be taken as final and definitive?

One way to approach this dilemma is to avoid specific treatments and decisions and deal only with general attitudes and preferences. However, Lockhart et al (2001) demonstrate the complexity of this process also, and point out that we do not yet have consensus on what is an acceptable level of stability of judgement. In their own study, they found that individuals' ratings of 'states worse than death' changed quite significantly over time, particularly their rating of the most serious health conditions as their own health declined. As the authors point out, this means that if an earlier advance directive were followed by medical practitioners, patients with diminished mental capacity or serious communication problems might be denied aggressive treatment when they do not wish to have their death hastened. Similarly, loss of mental capacity is one of the states most frequently cited as one in which people would not wish to continue. From personal observation in close contact with persons with dementia over a period of years, I would suggest that they do not necessarily experience their life in its late stages in the negative terms which they might have feared at an earlier stage. The same cannot usually be said for the carers, however – and therein lies one of the major dilemmas about whose wishes and decisions should be paramount.

Informal carers

Evidence that most deaths follow an extended period of increasingly intensive care and that the presence of an informal carer is a key variable in whether or not death occurs at home (Klinkenberg et al, 2005) leads us into one other very important aspect of death in old age. Many of the deaths in old age involve not just one central person, but two. The increasingly common pattern of spouse or partner caring, where caring and dependency are reciprocal and the balance shifting, is a significant feature of ageing and no small contributory element in our health and social care systems. Moreover, a related factor of people living longer is that adult offspring, caring for an aged parent, may themselves have reached old age. The angle of the older carer adds a significant dimension which should be taken into account when considering the care of the dying older person. That aside, primary carers are crucially important to those dying at home, both in enabling some to actually die in their own home and in enabling many more to stay at home for as long as possible, until their ultimate decline. When the older person does enter residential or nursing home care, it is not uncommon for the informal carer, particularly when this is the partner, to spend a large part of each day at the care home and to continue to carry out some caring tasks. In specialist palliative care services as well, the role of the carer may be crucial. Much of the innovation, especially in northern Europe, is to be found in home hospice schemes whose success largely depends on the active involvement of an informal carer. In the Longitudinal Aging Study Amsterdam, 80 per cent of those who had died of cancer had died at home, in marked contrast to those who had died of other causes (Klinkenberg et al, 2005).

Some older carers have expressed concerns about this transfer of responsibilities from professionals in what they see as a skilled activity requiring training. For younger carers, even those over 60, caring for someone who is dying is not necessarily something which they have observed or experienced before, and for the older age groups, its intensity may be beyond their physical and mental capabilities. There was a suspicion in the Sheffield study that encouraging carers to look after dying older relatives was a means of denying older people specialist medical care. At the same time, they were ambivalent about strangers taking over the bodily care of a loved one, fearing the process becoming impersonal and the importation of technology and night-time professional support turning their home into a hospital (Seymour, 2003).

However, perhaps the most difficult and least understood caring situation arises from the lack of recognition that this older person is in the dying stage of life, because they do not have a terminal diagnosis. Yet the common pattern for carers of people with dementia, Parkinson's disease and stroke survivors, for example, is that they become progressively more involved in giving personal and 'nursing' care, with varying degrees of help and perhaps interspersed with periods of respite care or hospitalisation, until some critical health event results in the final admission and death in hospital. Just occasionally, as in the sympathetic account provided by a daughter and granddaughter, *Living with Mother – Right to the Very End* (M. Hanson, 2006), the family system manages to care for the older person so that they die at home. Hanson's account gives us a rare insight into the fluctuating surprises and disappointments of a continuing relationship with someone who is affected by the physical and mental deterioration which might be expected in very old age. We have, however, little formal knowledge about the dying of older people in the community, for all the research and policy and practice initiatives aimed at enabling people to continue living in their own homes for as long as possible.

The needs of these carers are considerable, and in the UK formally recognised in legislation, but what is little recognised is that they are actually caring for someone who is dying and the implications of that. In my own study of people with Parkinson's disease and their carers, it was those carers who were giving both night-time and nursing care, often in poor health themselves, who indicated a significant impact on their emotional well-being and were most likely to say that they were not sure how much longer they could carry on (Holloway, 2006b). A Swedish study (Larson et al, 2005) developed four sub-scales – 'worries', 'powerlessness', 'personal adjustment' and 'social isolation' – in their questionnaire tool for understanding the life of spouse carers following a partner's stroke. Gonzalez-Ramos provides us with a poignant account of her elderly father ending the life of his wife before committing suicide (Gonzalez-Ramos, 2000). Most carers, however, have to negotiate the transition from caring for a dying older person, to mourning their loss.

Bereavement and grief in old age

This is a book about death, but it cannot go unremarked that old age is commonly characterised by a range of losses – physical, emotional, material – as well as loss through death (Scrutton, 1995; Thompson, 2002). Sometimes it is the cumulative effect of these losses which makes bereavement particularly hard to bear. Sometimes it is the other losses attending the bereavement on which the grief becomes focused. Moreover, it should be remembered that dying brings with it losses which are grieved by the dying person. Nevertheless, as Raphael (1984, p 285) reminds us, dying and bereavement in old age may bring 'grief of a gentler kind', in part because there has been opportunity to anticipate the loss and also because the death of a significant person in the older person's life will normally have been preceded by bereavements at a younger age.

This approach to understanding bereavement in old age has, however, all too frequently resulted in health and social care professionals ignoring the effect of grief on the older person, and of other, younger family and friends misunderstanding their behaviour. So, for example, assessments are made of the mental and physical functioning and everyday coping skills of the older person, which ignore the fact that grieving persons often experience confusion, forgetfulness and extreme fatigue, and neglect self-care. Family members become frustrated or upset by hostile, uncooperative and generally 'difficult' behaviour because they fail to understand that a range of irrational responses, including anger and anxiety, are a normal part of grief, as much for the older person when the death is 'expected' as for the younger bereaved person dealing with an untimely death. A number of writers have suggested that both dying and bereavement are not necessarily easier in old age (Lund, 1989b; Williams, 1990; Jecker and Schneiderman, 1994). Others suggest that the predominant approach which assumes that death will be greeted with equanimity, even relief, in old age, is another example of the ageism which pervades society and is reflected in the attitudes of the providers of health and social care as much as anyone else (Moss and Moss, 1989; Morgan, 1995).

Theories of dying and bereavement

Contemporary diversification in theorising about bereavement and grief is all to the good where older people are concerned, since the early seminal work, such as Lindemann's (1944) work following the Boston nightclub fire disaster, might be presumed to have limited application to bereavement in old age given the rather different patterns of older people's dying. A number of features of theories which assume the necessity of 'breaking bonds' and moving through stages in both dying and grief are problematic when transposed on to these experiences in old age. For example, the final stage of grief usually involves the notion of 'recovery' and reinvestment in life – in fact, Worden's original formulation of the tasks of mourning suggests that the final task is to 'withdraw emotional energy and reinvest it in another relationship' (Worden, 1982, p 15). Scrutton, in a determined attempt to counter ageist attitudes, which assume that older people are no longer interested in life and merely waiting for death, suggests a number of ways in which the older bereaved person can be helped to re-engage and reinvest socially, including making new relationships (Scrutton, 1995). There is an underlying assumption that a person who fails to do so is unhelpfully 'stuck' in grief. While a degree of social reinvestment may or may not be desirable and feasible for a person who has lost a partner in their 60s, we cannot avoid the fact that for a person in their 80s or 90s, who has lost a lifelong partner, whose health is failing and whose social world has drawn in as a result, 'reinvestment' may be neither desired nor practical. On the other hand, such people will recount with pleasure (to a sympathetic listener) a continuing sense of their deceased partner's presence and the comfort afforded by carrying on daily 'conversations'. This does not necessarily mean that they have given up on life, as Amy Hanson's poignant and funny glimpses of life with her 96-year-old grandmother indicate:

> I didn't know whether to laugh or cry as I passed her room today. Through the gap in the door I saw this old lady, sitting on the commode … She cannot read any more so the mobile library brings her story tapes. I can hear one now … 'Wow, I'm dizzy,' Nell said, breathless now. 'I felt a tingling inside, not unpleasant. Almost like you do when you're thinking – really thinking – about sex.' And I'd thought she was sitting there thinking about death. (A. Hanson, 2006)

We should not rule out the possibility either, that the younger widow or widower may neither wish to replace their partner nor add to their existing social contacts and continue to engage with life whilst cherishing that significant bond. Field found ample evidence in the recordings of older people for the Mass Observation Project in England of the importance of continuing memories in ongoing life (Field, 2000). The notion that 'I am the person I am now at least in part because of that relationship and therefore I still have that person' is one which I as a counsellor and researcher have heard variously expressed many times. The recent work on memorials and contemporary memorialisation practices (see Chapter Seven) provides us with many examples of the ways in which older people in particular perpetuate the relationship with a significant person after death, as a means of carrying on with life. Indeed, many have not experienced adult life, to any significant degree, without that person. The theory of 'continuing bonds' offers a theoretical understanding which may be more sympathetic to the experience of bereavement in old age, where the length and sometimes exclusive intensity (at least latterly) of the relationship may be its defining features.

The assertion of a death-denying society appears to hold good when it comes to old age. The older person, particularly the very old and confused, may be excluded from family discussions about the illness of a relative or friend and the death may be kept from them. Sometimes it is simply the case that no one thinks to keep them informed. For the older person in institutional care, a number of studies have shown the efforts made by staff in residential and nursing care homes to conceal the death of a resident from the others, and to fail to inform those known to be friends of the severity of the illness, and eventual death, of their friend. Still less are efforts made to enable them to participate in the funeral, visit and make memorials or to recognise and listen to their grief (Philpott, 1989; Hockey, 1990; Komaromy, 2000; Franklin et al, 2006). There are of course some exceptions to this general pattern: Komaromy points out that the Catholic homes in her study were careful to provide the opportunity to pay respects to the body, and Chapter Seven discusses the practice of parallel funerals for people too frail or sick to attend the actual event.

Loss of the relationship is not the only loss experienced when a significant person dies, however. It is often the accompanying losses which are the complicating factors for an older person and which are the principal mediators of bereavement in old age. Loss of a significant person in old age may mean loss of all companionship, any regular social contact, their mediator with the outside world, financial security, and finally bidding farewell to sexual expression. The particular feature of bereavement in old age is not that any or all of these are inevitable, nor that they are confined to bereavement in old age, but that the physical and social circumstances of old age make the older bereaved person particularly vulnerable to these attendant losses and they represent considerable risks to their quality of life. Unlike the person who has died, however, they are not for the most part irreplaceable. Much can be achieved by family, friends and formal service providers helping the older person to replace elements of their life that have been lost, without which they may be at risk of depression and self-neglect. Summarising the key findings from a number of studies of older bereaved spouses, Lund (1989b) states that social support could be said to be moderately helpful in helping the older person to adjust to life without their spouse. It was, however, the *quality* of the relationships and opportunities for contact that determined the extent to which they contributed to the older person's adjustment, not the number or type of contacts.

Widowhood

Arriving at the state of widowhood is generally reckoned to be one of the key social transitions in all societies. As a social state it is one that is crucially constructed by gender. As a result, much of the focus has been, and will continue to be, on widows. Many bereavement studies present a bleak picture of older widows, their primary status in adult society removed, their identity one that is problematic for them and those around them and their socioeconomic position fragile (for example, Williams, 1990; Parkes, 1996) – what Martin-Matthews, reflecting on the penchant for remarriage in old age, describes as being 'one man away from poverty' (Martin-Matthews, 1999). However, Martin-Matthews also provides us with a very useful picture of how widowhood is changing, not least being the fact that the increase in divorce leaves many more people, including men, single, their social networks disrupted, increasing numbers childless and, in essence, experiencing the most isolated experience of 'bereavement'. Demographic change has resulted in a decline in the incidence, but increase in the prevalence, of older widows. This in itself, however, may be leading towards a different experience of widowhood, particularly for women, in contemporary society.

Much depends, of course, on the personal and social circumstances of the older woman at the time of her bereavement, including, importantly, her health and the degree to which she may have been exhausted and socially isolated by a long period of caring (Burton et al, 2006). Nevertheless, the commonly recognised phenomenon of personal growth occurring through coping with bereavement appears to be particularly evident in studies of older widows. Silverman (2007) documented the transformatory aspects of widowhood occurring through involvement in self-help organisations and Matthews' work demonstrated the importance of friendship for older women's quality of life (Matthews, 1986). This makes it even more important for service providers to recognise the friendships formed by older women in residential care and hence their experiences of bereavement when another resident dies. The knowledge that some older widows find a new lease of life should also lead service providers to encourage this positive attitude in the older woman temporarily debilitated by grief.

Untimely dying

Lund (1989) points out that the cumulative evidence does not suggest that being able to anticipate the loss affects older people's process of adjustment after a bereavement, one way or the other. A more recent study, however, of 193 bereaved older spouses, found that an unexpected death put them at risk of depression (Burton et al, 2006). Most professionals who provide services to older people will be familiar with the scenario in which the 'wrong one' in a partnership dies first. This may be the person who as the least frail carried the caring responsibility for the other, or it may be that in the assumptions the couple had always made in their relationship, the other one was supposed to 'go first'. For the surviving older person in these situations, the affects of grief such as anger and disbelief may be strongly evident.

A further complication of bereavement in old age for older people in the twenty-first century, is that the picture of timely, natural death, with the older person learning to cope through a number of bereavements over a period of time, may not necessarily hold. The fact that many people now live into very old age potentially creates a degree of untimeliness. So some parents will outlive children who have themselves reached middle or late adulthood, only to then succumb to accident or disease, such as cancer. The shock and existential challenge of such a loss are likely to be profound for the surviving aged parent. Moreover, such family members may have been relied upon for support and a series of accompanying losses (as discussed above) follows. In the reverse situation, although the death of the aged parent is the natural order of things, the son or daughter may themselves have reached old age without previously experiencing a significant bereavement. It cannot be presumed that knowledge that the mother's or father's 'time had come' necessarily removes the impact of the reordering of one's 'place', which occurs when a parent dies. Likewise, the gradual loss of siblings, especially when these are younger and also when one is the last surviving of a generation, may provoke a grief reaction, which is all too often ignored or misunderstood by those around the older person. Such grief reactions may be further complicated in an older person who experiences short-term memory loss, but whose long-term recall is clear. Experiencing and accepting the 'reality of the loss' may be as painful as if the bereavement had occurred at a much younger age.

Dementia and grief

Relatively little attention has been paid to understanding grief as experienced by the person with dementia. In fact, as has often been the case in health and social care, it is the practitioner literature which appears to be leading the way, but doing so on the basis of some intuitive leaps into therapeutic interventions. The empirical base for these is largely lacking. Some attempts have been made to transfer work with people with learning disabilities (for example, Oswin, 1991) into understanding grief in people with dementia (for example, Lewis and Trzinski, 2006) but this seems to me to be theoretically flawed. Much of the problem in helping someone with dementia to deal with their grief lies in the patchy nature of their memory and the fluctuating levels of their understanding of current events. Nevertheless, any attempts to take seriously and respond to the grief of a person with dementia are to be welcomed. Sheldon (1997) points out that there is now greater appreciation of the potential levels of awareness in people with dementia and therefore practitioners should proceed with the intention of communicating the simple facts of the death, supporting the older person, and encouraging their family, so that they can be as involved in meaningful events as they are physically able.

A number of practice initiatives have been described which the authors suggest are helpful. For example, Mackay (1993) suggests that offering reassurance that the dead person is at peace will reduce anxiety, although others suggest that as dementia advances, the older person does not have the level of cognitive functioning necessary to understand the concept of death (Rentz et al, 2004–5). In fact, the more specialist therapies, such as the 'space retrieval' and 'group buddies' interventions described by Lewis and Trzinski (2006), are said to be appropriate for the person with mild or early-stage dementia. 'Space retrieval' is a technique which provides new information, then tests recall at intervals, the intervening periods being concerned with other information or activity. Lewis and Trzinski describe how, when used with individuals with dementia who have experienced a bereavement, the fresh grief diminishes from session to session. This approach is targeting the problem that each time the information is given to people with dementia they tend to receive it as if for the first time. 'Group buddies' uses a relatively untested approach of transferring play therapy techniques, as used with children, to group work with adults with cognitive and communication impairment. In this situation, the 'buddy' provides the physical and emotional security and the modelling behaviour for the expression of grief.

It is important to remember in all these approaches that older people with dementia have developed the emotional and social maturity of an adult and have a lifetime of memories. The problem is that these may not be accessible to their helpers and we do not know to what extent they are operating at any given point for them. However, our approach should be to facilitate that adult functioning as far as possible. Benbow and Quinn (1990) describe how planned visits to the grave accompanied by a trusted helper can gradually help the older person with dementia to accept that the person has gone and to express their sadness. I myself recall a 90-year-old man who had severe dementia, breaking down and sobbing when reminded suddenly of his deceased brother. The experience seemed cathartic and to achieve completion of the emotional task, begun some years earlier when he himself, although frail and in the early stages of dementia, had spoken at the funeral. These behaviours and reactions are as we might observe in any grieving person. Undoubtedly, however, we need to add to our knowledge and understanding of grief experienced by the person with dementia. Given that around half of dementia sufferers are in institutional care (Jolley and Baxter, 1997), where it is doubtful how much attention is paid to the grief of residents generally, and that the dominant models of grief counselling rely on a cognitive approach, we may have a long way to go before people with dementia have their needs recognised and receive a sympathetic response.

Rather more attention has been paid to the grief experienced by the carers of people with dementia. This is on two counts, both during care-giving, as the 'person' they had always known may seem increasingly lost to them, and after the death, when caring ceases. The grief associated with caring for someone with dementia with whom one has had a close relationship, particularly that of partner, is now recognised to be complicated by the person both remaining and having, in some senses, 'gone' (Boss, 1999). In the first place, the carer themselves may not acknowledge that it is grief that they are experiencing, and classic signs such as anger, guilt and depression become subsumed into the general stress of caring and the frustration experienced by the restrictions placed on both parties' lifestyles. The cumulative losses, which may accelerate as the disease progresses, such as loss of communication, intimacy, a social life, emotional support and independence (for both parties) are not themselves recognised and thus the needs of the carer in these areas are neither acknowledged nor appropriately addressed. So, for example, a carer may feel unable to relinquish their partner to respite care, not because their sense of duty is such that they cannot allow themselves a break, but because to see their partner struggling in that unfamiliar environment, looked after by service providers who have no knowledge of the person who used to be, brings home the reality of the carer's loss and their grief is overwhelming. Adams and Sanders (2004) found that indications of grief, and depression linked to grief, were considerably more marked in carers of people in advanced stages of dementia than in those caring for people in the early stages, and this, of course, is precisely the stage when the couple are likely to need formal services the most.

Marwit and Meuser (2005) point out the escalating scale of this problem for twenty-first century healthcare systems, where this type of carer distress and the problems which ensue from such complicated grieving, in a population some of whom are themselves vulnerable through age and frailty, is likely to lead to further health problems. The authors have developed an inventory for measuring grief in carers of people with dementia, and identify its main 'clinical potential' as being the therapeutic benefits of the carer recognising their own feelings and having those feelings validated by external acknowledgement. Finally, although the death of a person with dementia can be anticipated, the 'liminal phase' discussed earlier in this chapter may be quite prolonged. Moreover, caring in situations of high stress has in itself been found to be a predictor of depression in bereavement (Burton et al, 2006), yet the common response of those around the bereaved carer is that the death must have come as a relief.

Conclusion

If this chapter has presented a picture of old age which appears to feed into ageist assumptions that 'it's downhill all the way', this was not the intention. It does, however, present a cumulative picture of physical deterioration, social discrimination, emotional hurdles and existential dilemmas for which today's older people and the societies they inhabit – albeit for many on its margins – are ill-prepared. This represents a considerable challenge for those charged with delivering the health and social care, which both holds death at bay and must shepherd towards it. The point has often been made, that today's old have experienced more death, routine and traumatic, than any previous generation (and this probably holds true across the developed and developing worlds). Yet their experiences and perspectives are possibly the least studied. This chapter has also shown that older people have a lot to contribute to understanding death and the reactions of human beings to it, but that their potential capacity to negotiate the difficult terrains of dying and bereavement often outstrips the resources at their disposal.

In all respects, dying in old age is both the majority dying and the disadvantaged dying. Health and social care services, including palliative care, are only just beginning to recognise this fact. The experience of bereavement is possibly the commonest significant life event in old age. Thus our understanding of quality of life at the end of a long life must also be about quality of dying and quality support for those who live through this phase with the older person.

Key questions for practitioners

1. Has this older person with whom I am working experienced a significant bereavement in old age? If so, are they acknowledged as a mourner? What are the attendant losses for this person?
2. Have I taken account of the impact of grief on behaviour and functioning in my assessment of this older person?
3. Is there a significant/unresolved loss in their past history which is impacting on their current emotional state/care planning decisions?
4. If there is a current bereavement, is the older person who survives included in/excluded from making arrangements and participating in the funeral, burial/cremation and memorial events? Does this older person need support in order to participate?
5. Do I make time to listen to the thoughts and feelings of this older person about their own dying, the care of people close to them, their experiences of loss? Are there indicators that they might need particular help and should I refer them to someone else?
6. If this older person is dying, are they getting appropriate care? Is attention paid to their individual wishes, especially if communication is difficult? Are they given the same opportunities to prepare for their death as a younger person?
7. How might their cultural/religious background frame their dying/bereavement experience and can I facilitate their drawing on these resources?

Note

[1] More commonly known in the UK as DNRs – do not resuscitate orders.

SEVEN

The aftermath of death

Introduction

One of the points this book is trying to get across is that beliefs and practices surrounding death and dying are in a state of flux. Possibly one of the areas which is changing most is our approach to marking the end of life. Funerals, and all that surrounds them, are increasingly the subject of comment and debate and it seems that very little is as predetermined as may have been the case for previous generations. In order to make some sense of the burgeoning literature, both scholarly and popular, and to consider the implications of these changes for professionals working alongside people affected by a recent (and maybe not so recent) death, it may be helpful to separate out the various processes and events.

First, we are dealing with a number of public events (even the private ceremony is to some extent a public event), principally the funeral, burial, cremation and memorial service or gathering. Second, these events are controlled by society through legislation, municipal policies and cultural norms. The body must be formally released for burial, and there are controls on where it may be buried and what sort of memorial may be erected.[1] The celebrant, whether a religious minister or secular officiant, will be guided by their own tradition and culture as to the content of the funeral. Particular religions may have rules about the timing of burial and preparation of the body. Third, the events through which we mark and deal with the end of life are constructed as social acts and to a large extent circumscribed by a mixture of cultural requirement and social convention. The changing nature of the public face of death can only be understood in the light of broader social and cultural change. Fourth, as social acts, funerals provide the vehicle for phenomena which sociologists refer to as commemoration, disposal and memorialisation. However informal the character of the occasion, there is, nevertheless, some ceremonial element, in which a degree of stylised expression is used – often described in terms of rite, ritual and symbolism. Belonging to the act of memorialisation are the artefacts of private graves, war memorials, plaques, benches, and other 'permanent' memorials, which have been of huge interest to social historians and anthropologists. Increasingly, we are seeing a wide range of transitory memorials (such as roadside flowers) which may be periodically renewed in repeated acts of remembrance.

Fifth, funerals and memorials are not just social and corporate acts. These social acts have particular individual significance and impact. The social rituals and symbols associated with them also provide for the individual experiences of parting, acknowledging loss and marking social transition. In contemporary society it is the emotional state of individual mourners that is often of prime concern. Attending, or perhaps actively participating in, the funeral, involves the bereaved individual or family in a social act laden with cultural overtones at the same time as they are experiencing emotional, psychological and spiritual trauma. In a society of cultural pluralism, shifting attitudes to the body and 'customised' beliefs and spiritual practices, it is hardly surprising that we see some bereaved people alienated by a traditional funeral which apparently failed to reflect the essence of the person who has died or to reach the core needs of those who are left, whilst others are bewildered and floundering as they try to choose their own 'right' form of commemoration. Yet research has repeatedly noted the importance of the funeral in the mourning process and hence the longer-term adjustment of bereaved people. Aries has described the nobility from the middle ages to the late nineteenth century as 'presiding' over their own deaths, reaching beyond the deathbed to dictate the funeral and burial arrangements (Aries, 1974). The twentieth century also saw the large public event extended beyond the state funeral for royalty and political heads of state to globally and nationally recognised celebrity persons. The emotional engagement with such funerals of large numbers of people is another significant feature of late modernity, as is the practice of replicating in their own ceremonies choice of music, poems and the like. Engaging together in planning their funeral and what should happen to their body, has become an important part of 'dying well' for many people and their families in contemporary society.

Funerals

The early formulations of the modern death thesis examined in Chapter Three placed some emphasis on the demise of the modern funeral. While still an act of commemoration, the reduction in ritual and reducing of the funeral to a relatively brief and sparse ceremony was seen to have contributed to the inhibiting of mourning. Nevertheless, the funeral continued to be seen as an important marker in the grief process, its function being in the main to bring home the reality of the death. The emphasis was very much on the individual's process of adjustment rather than focusing on the funeral itself. Very little was added to this picture until the recent explosion of interest in funerals as events, with mourners seeking to replace the traditional funeral as conceived in western Christendom.

A parallel development has been the burgeoning funeral industry, in which interest was first aroused by Jessica Mitford's treatise entitled *The American Way of Death* (Mitford, 1963). Mitford mounted a powerful and emotive attack on 'greedy' funeral directors, who she saw as taking advantage of the vulnerability of bereaved relatives, selling services which they did not want and turning the whole process of death into a grotesque parody of the American lifestyle. Mitford was concerned to expose the business practices of a funeral industry which she saw as trading on the desire of Americans to control and prettify death and take away its horror. Mitford sparked off an interest in the American funeral industry which was not until much later mirrored in the UK (Howarth, 1996; Office of Fair Trading, 2001). However, her analysis has been contested. Laderman (2003) argues that, although there had been critics before of the growing influence and authority of funeral directors, particularly from ministers of religion who saw their role as pastors and meaning-makers being appropriated, the American funeral industry was merely making provision for what contemporary Americans want. Although Laderman himself has been criticised (Stearns, 2004), there is growing consensus that changes in funeral practices in contemporary society reflect a consumerist society which privileges individual customised choices over handed-down traditions.

This emphasis on the dying and bereaved as consumers is reflected in the UK, where organisations to regulate the industry and an Office of Fair Trading inquiry (OFT, 2001) all demonstrate a concern that information should be easily accessible and services provided in such a way that choices can be made in the absence of high-pressure selling. The implicit theme in the background academic report to the inquiry (Johnson et al, 2001) is that contemporary mourners are disorientated, confused and reliant on funeral service providers to guide them through a process for which they have little useful experience and no automatic given structure. Littlewood showed from her 1980s' research that many mourners felt disappointed by the traditional funeral they had arranged, and alienated from its religious rites. They had expected assistance in their quest to find meaning in their bereavement, but had instead found the funeral an ordeal with which they were unable to connect emotionally or spiritually (Littlewood, 1992).

Funeral ritual and mourning

The study of ritual is a useful starting point in seeking to understand contemporary funerals and trends in commemoration, disposal and memorialisation. Anthropologists argue that the funeral performs a number of functions to do with the living taking their leave of the dead. The prolongation of these rituals beyond the funeral event is referred to as *mourning*. Once again, the work of Hertz provides us with a theoretical framework for understanding these rituals, which Metcalfe and Huntington (1979) and, much later, Walter (1994) have organised into a triangle of essential elements: the body, or corpse; the living, or mourners; and the soul, or dead entity. Both adaptations discuss the funeral as a means of representing the interests of each and performing the rituals necessary to each. Metcalfe and Huntington are also concerned with the relationships between them. Thus, the mourners, as the living, must disassociate from the dead, as both corpse and social person, and the relationship between the corpse and its disposal, and the soul (or dead entity) and its ongoing journey, must be represented. In contemporary funerals, however, there is broad agreement that the function of the funeral has moved towards performing the rituals essential for only one element of the triangle – the mourners – although Parkes does argue that the modern funeral remains to some extent the gift of the bereaved to the deceased (Parkes, 1996).

Fear of the dead

There is considerable agreement among anthropologists that a significant number of rites attached to funerals provide evidence of the fear engendered in the living by the dead. This results in both attempts to appease the dead and in their open rejection (Grainger, 1998). Much of Hertz's essay (1907) dealt with explanations for this fear engendered in the living. The idea that the living, particularly close relatives, are contaminated by their contact with the dead and must adopt a new identity is common in a number of religions and cultures. Rituals may appear to simultaneously *approach* the world of the dead person, for example by placing food and clothing with the corpse, and to *separate* from that world by focusing on new life and regeneration. In Hertz's explanations, these behaviours emanate from a desire to appease the dead, so that they will leave the living alone, and to render the dead harmless by assisting them in their passage towards their new state or destination. A sociohistorical explanation for these rituals is that the departed spirit is potentially dangerous and threatening of the social order. Bloch and Parry (1982) argue that the funeral ceremony 'involves the reassertion of society', in which 'the collective consciousness of the living has been resettled by the funerary rituals' (p 4).

At first sight, it may be difficult to see any reflection of these beliefs in contemporary western culture and funeral ritual. Aside from the occasionally-heard saying, 'Don't speak ill of the dead' – presumably reflecting folklore about wandering malevolent spirits – fear of the dead seems not to feature in our ritual. However, close examination of the Christian funeral ritual, and of pre-rituals such as the administration of 'last rites', reveals considerable anxiety about the dead and about the state of being dead, from the living. A Christian funeral service, whether expressed through formal liturgy or free worship, turns attention away from the crumbling mortal remains and focuses on the hope of resurrection and eternal life, all the while assuring those who are left behind that the deceased person is commended to the love and mercy of God. The sacraments administered to the person close to death are similarly concerned to offer forgiveness and reconciliation, and the focus of the pastoral task is to facilitate the individual making their own peace and preparing for the next stage of their 'journey' (Ainsworth-Smith and Speck, 1982). Thus pre-funeral and funeral rites can be seen as an attempt to 'tame' the threat of death and to facilitate a comfortable relationship between the living and the dead.

Can the same function be observed in the 'ritual' of the increasingly popular secular funerals and the customised, usually secular, touches which relatives and friends frequently add to the funeral service? Our knowledge of these is still largely anecdotal but observations would suggest that they are predominantly life-affirming and celebratory (for example, playing a favourite or significant piece of music). It is possible that celebrating and affirming the life in the face of death, without connection to any belief system concerning a life hereafter, is nevertheless an act of asserting the pre-eminence of life over death and warding off its threat to those that remain.

Separation from the dead

The other important function which is consistently reproduced in funeral ritual has to do with separating from the dead, expressed in some cultures as rejection of the dead and in others as 'letting go'. Grainger (1998) describes a number of rituals which amount to symbolic dismissal of the deceased person and others which underline the irreversibility of death, the fact that the person who has died has 'crossed over to the other side' (such as sealing the entrance to a tomb so that the person may not return). This particular piece of symbolism is the one most often taken up by modern therapists, who argue for the catalystic value of the funeral in helping the bereaved to accept the reality of the death and engage with their grieving (Manning, 2001; Worden, 2003). Thus the revivalist movement emphasises the cathartic value of the funeral ceremony, in facilitating expression of the emotions associated with the loss and letting go of a loved one. Some sociologists, however, are dismissive of this type of activity as ritual, arguing that the sharing of personal feelings does not substitute for, nor perform the functions of, a social ritual (Walter, 1994). Since contemporary funerals and memorial services increasingly incorporate personal customised elements, there is an important issue at stake here. The universality of death rituals appears to demonstrate that human beings have an enduring need to develop behaviours and symbols which publicly grapple with the meaning of death. In late modernity, it seems that we need to infuse that social ritual with a personal meaning which the prescribed forms do not necessarily facilitate. The problem lies in how to find the forms through which to give shared social meaning to personal experience. There are limited examples of this being achieved, for example where a young person's school cohort remembers their friend through a code of dress, badge or choice of music which was and is significant for the group to which the dead youngster belonged.

The traditional funeral

If the function of the funeral is to commemorate the person who has died and secure their separation from the living and transition into the state of being dead, then its content must be meaningful for those attending. For the follower of a particular religion, a large part of the content of the funeral service is provided for them. As yet we have little information about how well this religious symbolism is understood by most people who currently choose a religious funeral. In my own research undertaken in 1991 into the spiritual and philosophical frameworks employed by dying and bereaved persons (Lloyd, 1996), the most commonly recognised Christian symbols concerned the dualism of the physical, mortal body, which is thrown off and left behind, and the immortal soul which proceeds to an afterlife and with which the living may continue to connect on some level (this was not always expressed in peaceful terms). This need for 'spiritual proximity' appears to mirror the need for social proximity, which anthropologists have argued is one of the functions of memorialisation (Kellaher et al, 2005) and emotional proximity, which grief therapists have explored extensively in their search for therapeutic techniques which enable the grieving person to complete 'unfinished business'.

Emke (2002) also records the fact that anecdotal evidence suggests that in the western tradition there is now little emphasis on commending the deceased person to God's care, and that even among the clergy, the promise of the resurrection comes some way behind offering support for mourners and facilitating the grieving process. In his study of funeral practice in Newfoundland, Canada (which he emphasises is considerably more traditional and less secularised than most western communities), only 17.5 per cent of clergy respondents identified a theological purpose to the funeral service. Although not focusing specifically on the funeral service, my research a decade earlier had shown hospital and hospice chaplains in the UK to privilege secular counselling skills in their contacts with dying and bereaved people over any sort of religious or theological content, which some cited as unhelpful to mourners (Lloyd, 1995).

In addition to this downplaying of religious content, the traditional Christian funeral has been increasingly adapted and 'customised' to fit the wishes of individual families. Most commonly this takes the form of close mourners choosing, and maybe giving, particular readings or musical items. These may or may not have religious content although they will generally be on a broadly spiritual theme. Much depends here on the approach of the minister leading the service as to what they are happy to incorporate and maybe steer the family towards. The other main adaptation concerns a focus on the life and character of the person who has died. Historically, the funeral eulogy was a contentious matter and frowned upon by some religions. However, in our twenty-first-century cult of the individual, personalising the ritual is seen as good practice, and it is usual for the minister to gather information from the family in order to deliver a brief homily about the person who has died, or a member of the family or close friend will do this themselves. In a recent Belgian study, Vandenthorpe reported that old and new traditions are combining in the funeral service, with clergy welcoming greater involvement of the family (Vandenthorpe, 2000). Young and Cullen, in their study of death among East Londoners (Young and Cullen, 1996), decried the impersonal religious service often conducted by clergy and called for funerals to be made more personal as a primary need. Emke (2002) notes that over half of the clergy respondents in his Newfoundland study reported greater personalisation as one of the changes in funeral services which they had experienced in recent history.

Other forms of personalisation include choosing a hymn (or other piece of music), which was meaningful for the person who has died or for their relationship with one or more of the principal mourners. This personal customising is possibly the key adaptation of the traditional Christian funeral service over the last decade, and is an indication of widening secularising trends. However, the old and the new do not always sit harmoniously alongside each other. Moore and Phillips suggest that the fast pace of emerging death culture in the US does not meet the needs of many African-Americans, whose traditional rituals are rooted in their suffering history, and are crucial to black identity (Moore and Phillips, 1994).

Secular funerals

Ben-Amos, in his review of state funerals in France (Ben-Amos, 2000), notes that the 'great men' of the nineteenth-century French Republic, with their affirmations of secularism, secured their place in the collective 'immortality' and turned their funeral into a 'sacred' event by making it into a spectacular occasion, centred around their own achievements and standing in the community. There is much that resonates here in the secular funerals which have proliferated over the past decade in the formerly predominantly Protestant English-speaking and north European world. For a wealthy minority this may incorporate theatrical trappings which echo the nineteenth-century great man's funeral (Leland, 2006) but for most ordinary people it involves making the occasion 'special' rather than spectacular, special to that unique individual who has died and to the mourners' individual and collective memories.

In 1980 Miss Barbara Smoker, President of the National Secular Society, gave an address to the Cremation Society Conference (UK) on the subject of non-religious funerals. As one of the earliest secular officiants at funerals, she summarised the central tenets of the secular funeral as follows:

- that the funeral ceremony is solely for the benefit of the bereaved;
- that materialist beliefs nevertheless require a funeral out of respect for a unique human life;
- that it should provide for a review of the person's life;
- that it should allow mourners to share feelings of loss;
- that it should be a ceremony and provide the opportunity for ritual 'leave-taking' of the person who has died.

This framework for what we might term the 'mainstream' secular funeral has remained remarkably unchanged over the last 25 years. The change that has occurred is that such funerals have become commonplace and officiants are relatively easily available and themselves organised (Barbara Smoker did suggest that the ideal secular funeral is if a close family friend or even family member can lead the proceedings, but acknowledged that many do not feel able to do this. Anecdotal evidence suggests that this practice remains rare, most people preferring a formally designated person to officiate). The British Humanist Association, for example, has a register of officiants and offers published guidance for bereaved relatives planning a non-religious funeral. In Australia, 'secular celebrants' are well established and generally work through a standard process of contact and discussion with the family to develop the funeral content (Walter, 1989). Commonly, the pattern of the 'service' is very similar to a religious funeral, alternating readings and music, but without liturgy.

However, two crucial differences have emerged as a corollary to the religious–secular divide. First, the secular funeral has as its centrepiece the 'funeral biography' where the religious service has the funeral address (albeit these days usually incorporating a degree of biographical information). Second, there is an increasing and explicit trend for secular funerals to be life-affirming. Where the religious funeral deals, at least in liturgical form, with death as the great paradox of life, the secular funeral does not purport to dwell on these questions, although it may focus on the feelings of loss experienced by the bereaved. Ros Coward, writing in the *Guardian* newspaper, expresses the dilemma thus:

> A few years ago all the funerals I went to seemed to hit the wrong note. None of the dead had been churchgoers, so services were often excruciating.

But she goes on to say:

> DIY celebrations sometimes feel like parties, but with the main guest absent. Death here ceases to be the great leveller but another demonstration of that person's status, position and popularity. The modern need for consolation and celebration abandons the harshness of traditional rituals that can be infinitely more cathartic. (Coward, 2002)

Walter similarly points to the 'struggle to find words to express the universality of death, to express our anxiety about our own mortality', as a fundamental weakness of the secular funeral (Walter, 1989, p 399). The key to this, it is suggested, is the loss of traditional public ritual alongside the search for private customised rituals (Walter, 1994; Hockey, 2001). Gore, commenting on the replacement of customs such as drawn curtains, removal of hats and other indications of 'paying respects', with the facility for friends and neighbours to view the body in the funeral parlour, suggests that this is:

> for personal need, not as an act of support from the community to the family at home, thus eroding the community-based funeral support of the past and replacing local customs with distant attenuated ritual. (Gore, 2001, p 217)

'Alternative' funerals

No less important to fulfilling the functions of commemoration, separation and transition, is the form which the funeral takes. Recent years have seen a huge range of alternatives to the traditional funeral service. They are necessarily of a secular nature but distinguished from mainstream secular funerals by their non-traditional formats and practices. It is in some 'alternative' funerals that we see the life-affirming trend taken to its most extreme. Perhaps unsurprisingly, given the American funeral industry which Mitford described, most of these ideas and practices originate in the US. According to a study by the National Funeral Directors Association, 62 per cent of Americans would prefer a customised event, only 13 per cent opting for a traditional funeral service (cited in Loyalka, 2005).

The term 'alternative funeral' covers a huge range of practices and it is perhaps useful to categorise the approaches. The first category is the individually personalised 'DIY funeral'. Such funerals are really an extension of the personalising touches which we have observed in traditional religious and secular funerals. The idea is that anything which was personally significant for the person who has died can be incorporated into an individually designed ritual to let them take their leave of the living. It is my view that these have all the hallmarks of a ceremony and constitute examples of the process which Walter hypothesises is resulting in a 'revival' of death in postmodernity (Walter, 2004). Underlying this, is the fact that in customising the funeral in this way, mourners (and also the dead who may have set out in detail their funerary wishes before their death) are wresting back control from the professionals. The *New Natural Death Handbook* advertises itself as 'covering everything you need to know about arranging a funeral yourself' (www.diyfunerals.co.uk). In fact, DIY funerals are more about control of what takes place than actually doing everything for oneself. One entrepreneur in Houston, Texas, has established what he calls a 'funeral concierge service', which claims to get for the funeral consumer whatever personal touch they require (Leland, 2006). *The Dead Good Funerals Book* (Gill and Fox, 2004) provides examples such as the lorry driver who requested that his coffin be driven on a flat-bed lorry along his usual route, including a stop for tea at the lorry drivers' cafe.

These 'ceremonies' are not necessarily sombre affairs. Often they are deliberately light-hearted. This brings us to my second category, which takes the view that we should make death a celebration, indeed fun. Lynn Isenberg, author of the light-hearted novel *The Funeral Planner* (2005), and founder of a business designed to treat the funeral as an entertainment event, describes disco parties and envisages celebrity appearances in the future (Loyalka, 2005; Leland, 2006). Although such ideas may seem frivolous, and certainly not mainstream at the moment, it is interesting that the promoters link their ideas to other life transitions, such as marriage, arguing that death should be treated to a similar celebratory event. This is not necessarily such an 'alternative' idea. In New Orleans, the jazz funeral is the tradition, the tradition being that the jazz band performs first a sober ritual, moving into the celebratory occasion after the body has been buried. A traditional Jamaican funeral shares a similar celebratory theme. Isenberg hints at the creation of new rituals and symbols as she centres her funeral planning service around the 'tribute video', which she describes as a 'spiritual biography' (Leland, 2006).

The third category of alternative funeral, which I am loosely terming the 'technological funeral', covers a range of options, some frankly futuristic whilst others stem from the IT which is a normal part of everyday life. The option of online funerals through use of webcams for mourners who cannot attend the actual event is increasingly widely advertised by funeral services, but little is yet known about level of take-up (Roberts, 2004). However, as mourners gradually come to consist of computer-literate generations, and in a context in which separated families and friends increasingly use the internet to keep in touch, it is not fanciful to suggest that this will become a major alternative. Its function, enabling all mourners to participate, recognises what has long been documented, that bereaved persons who are separated by geographical distance from the death and aftermath events, often have difficulty accepting the reality of the death. Further, widespread televising of state funerals and evidence of the viewing figures for such transmissions, as well as the subsequent comment in the press about the sympathetic or otherwise coverage, suggest that such forms of distance engagement are meaningful for participants. A related but traditional form of funeral is the 'parallel funeral service', in which a sick or old person in institutional care is enabled to take part in a simple brief service conducted at their bedside, with perhaps other friends and professional carers also present (Wrapson, 1999). In similar fashion, the author recalls, as a hospital social worker, arranging for the female members of a Muslim woman's community to spend the afternoon around her bed while the men held the funeral service for her stillborn baby.

At the futuristic end of the scale, a small number of 'space burials' are reported to have taken place (Wikipedia reports 150 individual remains up to 2004). This procedure involves launching small samples of the cremated remains of a number of individuals into space as part of an existing rocket launch. As with other events for which the term 'alternative funerals' is used, the funeral itself is not necessarily a significant part of the whole process – indeed, the authors of *The Dead Good Funerals Book* (Gill and Fox, 2004) make the point that it is not necessary to have a funeral at all. For many who opt for the alternative route, it is the disposal of the body which is of prime concern.

Burial and cremation

What happens to the body after the ceremony of commemoration, sometimes referred to as the *disposal* of the body, is of great cultural and religious significance. Both the method of disposal and its final resting place are important. The two mainstream forms of disposal are burial and cremation. Both are strictly regulated in the laws of all civilised societies. In Britain and northern Europe, some 70 per cent of people currently are estimated to opt for cremation (Pharos International, 2004; BioCycle World, 2006). In the US, burial remains the favoured option, although numbers of cremations are increasing steadily, accounting for 26 per cent of all disposals in 2000 (National Funeral Directors Association, 2006). Practice in the non-Anglo-Saxon world is largely determined by the dominant religious grouping(s), although the form and symbolism of cremation may be quite different to the way in which cremation is understood and practised in the UK, for example. Davies and Guest point out that traditional Indian cremation as practised by Hindus and Sikhs, is vastly different, in terms of what it symbolises, to the modern cremation which developed in the western world. The former places great emphasis on the heat of the fire releasing the spirit from the flesh which it consumes, whereas the latter is largely a utilitarian process governed by technical and sanitary considerations (Davies and Guest, 1999). Underpinning belief systems are particularly important in determining whether the choice is for burial or cremation because of the way in which the body, and its symbolic value, are understood. I myself recall that the form filled out by the social worker admitting an older person to residential care in the 1970s required them to ask the question, 'Would you prefer burial or cremation?' – and finding an appropriate time and way to ask it was a key part of one's training!

Until relatively recently, cremation was frowned upon by all Christian and Judaic traditions as well as Islam, and burial continues to be required for Orthodox Jews and Muslims; the Baha'i faith also requires burial. However, as it became the choice for the majority of Britons in the 1960s, all the Christian denominations relaxed their attitude, treating it as a matter of individual preference. Burial continues to be favoured by practising Catholics, particularly if the funeral is preceded by a wake with open casket. The Jewish Reformed movement has also relaxed its attitude to cremation, although it continues to regard it as important that the 'body', whether the corpse or the ashes, is kept whole. Those religions that require whole body burial usually do so because of a belief in subsequent resurrection of the body, or because of a belief in a liminal period in which the soul remains in the body before continuing its journey. Even where there is no objection to cremation, disquiet is often expressed by funeral directors as well as religious leaders about some of the more novel ideas for disposal of the ashes which involve splitting the ashes, doubts also expressed by some lay people (Kellaher et al, 2005). Equally some respondents in the ashes study wanted their own ashes to be eventually mingled with those of their dead spouse, so as to bring about a physical reunion.

Ecological issues

There is increasing recognition that a number of aspects of both traditional burial and cremation are not eco-friendly (Ward, 2004; Brown, 2005). Coffins made from expensive hardwoods from endangered species designed to resist decomposition, or cheaper versions made from chipboard stuck together with pollutant glues, are in themselves recognised as environmentally destructive. This is especially the case in cremation, when they are burnt in a process which is itself, although regulated, polluting the environment (BioCycle World, 2006). As a result of this growing awareness, 'green funerals', often involving burial in a woodland site, are growing in popularity, especially in the UK. To be accepted for a woodland burial, materials used have to be biodegradable (for example a cardboard or wicker coffin or natural cotton shroud) and there should be no or minimal embalming using harmful chemicals, freezing or dry ice being used to preserve the body instead. Woodland burials have close links with 'New Age' spirituality in their origins, and for most people choosing this option, there seems to be a strong metaphysical significance. Often mourners are carrying out the wishes of the person who has died and sentiments such as returning to the earth and feeding the new life of a tree or shrub planted to mark the grave, are expressed. The theme of regeneration and new life arising out of death and decay, which Van Gennep (1960) identified, and which can be seen in the rites of the major world religions, is strongly evident in the values and beliefs underpinning woodland burial. It is even stronger in the most recent trend – composting. Founded by a Swedish environmentalist, Wiigh-Masak, the human compost movement has patented a process of freeze-drying then shattering the body to be reused as compost feeding the land and, if desired, a specific 'living memorial'. The emphasis is on a form of disposal which is both ecologically sound and spiritually meaningful.

There are in addition two stages in disposal which occur before and after the 'main event' of burial or cremation. These are the preparation of the body before disposal, and disposal of the ashes. Both are richly imbued with ritual and symbolism.

Preparation of the body

Preparing the body for disposal is a universal procedure, required for both sanitary and social reasons. Indeed, the most dehumanising and degrading episodes in the history of humankind have involved public disrespect for the dead bodies of victims or enemies. In all cultures and throughout time, preparation of the body imbues the lifeless corpse with an identity linking it with the living. Mortuary ritual is thus concerned with the change from living person to dead body and the socially acceptable presentation of the corpse. In contemporary western culture, this often involves establishing a highly personal identity (for example, dressing in the colours of a sports team for a lifelong fan) and links with the personalising touches discussed in contemporary funerals.

These procedures are carefully prescribed, involving washing, laying out and dressing of the body. As with the symbolic practices already examined, these practical procedures are shaped by underpinning beliefs as well as being dictated by biological necessity. The overarching imperative is that the body should be made ready to take its leave of the living, and presentable for the living to relinquish the person to death. Each religious group, however, overlays these functions of washing, laying out and dressing with its own requirements concerning timing and order of events, appropriate persons to perform the various offices, and correct form of dress (see Green and Green, 1992, for a comprehensive description of the practices of different religious groups). There may be additional preferences concerning exact circumstances, such as location. These requirements have developed in each case because they stem directly from beliefs about what happens to the individual at death and after. Thus they are performed as rituals and it is extremely important to adherents to the faith that these rituals should be observed. In societies experiencing a decline in religious belief, there tends to be a corresponding relaxing of the ritual requirements. Thus, for example, Deeken points out that burial rites in Japan have become less elaborate as ancestor worship has declined, although as late as 1995 the Japanese paid five times as much for a funeral as Americans and eleven times as much as Britons (Deeken, 2004).

Considerable importance has been attached to what happens to the body, and the manner in which it is prepared, quite apart from any specific religious practice, however. So, for example, the development of stillbirth procedures in UK hospitals in the 1980s commonly included specific instructions to hospital staff to clean and wrap the dead baby before presenting her/him to the parents, as well as the taking of a photograph. Contained within this practice is a set of beliefs about the body and embodiment and the creation of a ritual to establish the stillborn child among the community of the living in order that the living might then relinquish the child. The author vividly recalls, as a hospital social worker, being asked to sort out a problem arising because nursing staff wished to prevent a mother having the photograph of her stillborn baby. At issue was the fact that, although the stillbirth procedure had technically been followed, it had not been done in such a way as to respect the implicit beliefs and values. An unwrapped baby, its disfigured face in full view, had been photographed next to an overflowing rubbish bin.

In Jessica Mitford's original exposé, the mortuary technician played a crucial role. Mitford described the popularity of elaborate embalming techniques, including suntans and makeovers. Such preparations of the body were seen by the 'modern death' analysts to belong to the death-denying culture of the twentieth century. Surprisingly, therefore, it is only in recent years, just as we have become more open about death, that we have seen a limited introduction in the UK of the 'prettifying' of the corpse in the American style (Howarth, 1996). Meanwhile, Lisa Cullen's recent investigation of the American way of death (Cullen, 2006) portrays a culture which has become increasingly inventive in its methods of preserving the physical remains, in parallel with a more casual openness about death manifested in the popularity of the TV series *Six Feet Under.* According to Cullen, this is not to so much to do with a denial of death as with a desire to control death.

If we return to our discussion of the inextricable intertwining of ritual practices and belief systems, however, this finding is not so surprising. The American funeral industry now explicitly targets its wares at the 'baby-boomer' generation. A youth-applauding culture has metamorphosed in the US, adapting to its ageing population, into an obsession with the 'ageless' body. Cosmetic surgery is commonplace and often extensive. In such a cultural context, it is not difficult to see that the person must present as well in death as in life. In fact, in a society where a whole raft of health promotion beliefs dictates lifestyle choices and everyday activities, it is entirely consistent for the dead body, with the intervention of the mortuary technician, to appear better than the individual in life. In the event of sudden death, caused by or causing trauma to the body, it must be restored not just to what it was, but sometimes to what it might have been. The UK has increasingly adopted this health and fitness agenda. If this hypothesis is valid, we may see more elaborate embalming techniques becoming more commonplace. However, the different language used in the US and the UK, where embalming is often referred to as 'sanitisation' (Green and Green, 1992), may be indicative of a different attitude to the process. If the priority is to stabilise the condition of the body while the arrangements for its disposal are made (and there may be circumstances which might cause delay such as a post-mortem and coroner's report) rather than to embark on a process of restoration so that the body might be presented in an open casket, then the practice will be limited to what is practically necessary. Davies (1996) argues that the popularity of cremation in the UK, whereas burial remains the most common method of disposal in the US, is closely related to the British tendency to 'hide' death. Therefore, rather than being ceremonially prepared, the body must be quickly reduced to next to nothing, a small pile of ashes. This argument is only sustainable, however, if all other rites and practices serve to hide death, and, as we have already seen, there is growing evidence that they do not, although they may seek to reaffirm life over death.

Preserving the body

Two contemporary methods of preparation do not lead to disposal through burial or cremation since they are themselves the method of disposal. The first is the practice of cryonics, which involves suspending the individual through freezing at death, in the hope that the technology will some day be developed to 'resurrect' them (this may be through cloning). Although limited in popularity and availability, cryonics has been around for some considerable time and might be seen as the ultimate expression of the human desire to control death. Cullen (2006) also investigated a process of mummification involving freezing as the last step. Interestingly, this is described by both providers and consumers in religious or spiritual terms, involving a long drawn-out funeral to assist the dead in their transition into another state, dictated by a 'spiritual will' made prior to death (sometimes a long time prior). The emphasis is on ritual to assist the dead, not the bereaved.

A more recent innovation is the practice of plastination (Walter, 2004; Cullen, 2006). Developed by a German anatomist named Gunther von Hagens, and initially confined to use in medical schools, the basic plastination involves replacing body fluids with a resin which hardens, thus permanently preserving the body in dry form. From 1996 onwards von Hagens mounted the Body Worlds public exhibitions, which toured internationally, displaying his 'plastinates' in a range of creative modes (for example, in particular physical poses or social identities). A small amount of research has been done on the impact of these displays on visitors, including their views on it as a method of disposing of the body (Walter, 2004).

While this can be reported as no more than indications of public reaction, a few points are worth noting. A surprising number of visitors expressed willingness to donate their bodies for plastination, and this seemed related to the extent to which the educational framework of the exercise was the primary impression. However, ethical and emotional issues were also raised, particularly when the exhibits appeared more person than anatomy. Cullen relays the disquiet expressed by the son of a Californian woman who has opted for plastination, because she has birthmarks which will make her recognisable and hence on display in death to those who knew her in life. To the woman herself, however, this is irrelevant, because, 'I define myself as spiritual … my identity is not in my body' (Cullen 2006, p. 135). While plastination is unlikely to become widely available or used as a method of disposal – for reasons of cost and space even if it achieved wide acceptance – it is an interesting illustration of where and how people draw the boundaries between the public and the private as well as the significance of the body and what it represents.

Disposal of the ashes

Another question concerns what happens to the ashes after cremation. It is interesting that although cremation itself has always been strictly regulated in law, what happens to the ashes afterwards is not, in the UK, although it is in the rest of Europe (Cook, 2006). This is leading to increasing calls for regulation by environmental agencies. The two main (and original) forms of disposal are containment in an urn, followed by interment or scattering. Interment of ashes is probably the closest approximation found in advanced societies to the secondary burial practices of more primitive cultures, although practical necessity is introducing a form of secondary burial in some societies. For example, both Hong Kong and Japan, experiencing a crisis in burial space, are introducing new secondary burial traditions. In Hong Kong, which already had the tradition of ossified remains being exhumed and kept in large jars, it is now possible to rent space in a funeral parlour for the cremated remains and a temporary shrine to be established, before moving to a more permanent site when space becomes available. In Tokyo, where there is an average of 30 applications for each public grave plot, legal restrictions on exhuming abandoned graves have been significantly eased so that the remains may be removed and deposited in communal graves. These practices are causing significant disquiet and leading to a marked move away from traditional funerary rituals led by monks to simple cremation and individually chosen modes of scattering the ashes (Rowe, 2003).

In the early popularisation of cremation in the UK, it was usual for the cremated remains to be collected without ceremony by the funeral director, and either interred or scattered in the Garden of Rest attached to the crematorium, or, in the earliest days, kept in a special building for the purpose (Davies and Guest, 1999). For many of the oldest old, this routine and somewhat impersonal procedure remains the norm today. However, both Davies and Guest (1999) and Kellaher et al (2005) point to a sharp increase in the number of bereaved collecting the ashes from the crematorium, reaching 56 per cent of all cremations by 2004 (Kellaher et al, 2005). There are only hazy statistics as to what happened to these sets of ashes, partly because it is known that people may scatter or bury ashes illicitly at family graves in order to avoid bureaucratic red tape and costly fees. As well as scattering or burying at a grave, common disposals are to scatter at a favourite outdoor location, including on water. At certain well-known beauty spots in the UK, this has been identified as an environmental hazard, with large quantities of ash solidifying, such that the Environment Agency has issued policy and practice guidelines to prevent further damage to the environment (Environment Agency of England and Wales, 2005).

The research undertaken in the 'ashes project' (Kellaher et al, 2005) has uncovered a huge range of individual practices, including keeping the ashes of a deceased spouse close by in the hope that they might eventually be reunited after death through the mingling of both sets of ashes. People chose the time, the place and the mode of disposal which felt right for them, and liked the idea of being in control of that process. However, there is also evidence from the popular media that bereaved people are often floundering as to what to do, and find themselves dealing with situations which take an unexpected turn, such as the ash blowing back in the mourners' faces, being spilt accidentally, and so on. Unsurprisingly, dark humour abounds. For some bereaved, however, these situations are deeply upsetting. The theme that runs through the accounts from Kellaher et al's respondents is that they needed to imbue meaning and their own forms of ritual into the disposal of the ashes. One family explained (Cook, 2006) that their relative had been on her way to the spot where they chose to scatter her ashes, and so they were 'completing the journey for her'.

Another common theme in the 'ashes project' research was the need for the bereaved to establish a focus for their mourning, often by marking the place where the ashes were buried or the spot where they were scattered, with some form of physical memorial. Sometimes, retaining the urn containing the ashes in the home served the same purpose. Lisa Cullen found other ways in her tour of current American death practices, of turning the ashes themselves into a permanent memorial, such as the production of a 'human diamond' from the remains.

Memorials

The process of memorialising the life that is gone, and the relationship which has been lost, is the final part of death's aftermath and it can be observed throughout history and across cultures. Memorials offer a form of immortality for those who have died as well as the possibility of a continuing link between those who have gone and those who remain. They may facilitate mourning or become fixed for the bereaved as substitutes for the person who has died or the shared life which is lost. As with commemoration and disposal, memorial practices in contemporary society are developing more diverse forms with considerable rapidity, and coexist alongside traditional forms. Memorials may be a concrete object (such as a gravestone), particular event (such as a memorial service) or ongoing activity (such as a memorial foundation). They may be a commonly shared type (such as the crematorium plaque) or informal and individually designed (although some of these, such as the placing of a bench or planting of a tree, are becoming so popular as to constitute 'new traditions'). They may be permanent (such as a stone monument) or transitory and renewable (such as flowers left by the roadside). They may mark the place of disposal, or not. The common thread running through all these forms of memorialising is that memorials provide a focus for social transition and a psychological and spiritual link between the living and the dead. One respondent in the author's research into spiritual and philosophical issues in dying and bereavement explained that he had retained his baby daughter's name as the password on his computer after she had died, commenting that he got something out of typing it in every time he used the computer (Lloyd, 1996).

Perhaps the most interesting feature of memorialising in the UK at present is the way in which these forms and traditions are combined, both by individuals and within communities. So, for example, a municipal cemetery may contain a huge variety of grave styles, ranging from the traditional headstone with a Protestant Christian cross and commonly worded inscription, to a completely personalised and secularised representation of the life of the deceased person, to a modern Buddhist shrine, to the colourful displays of plastic flowers more redolent of southern Europe.[2] Similarly, Reimers (1999) describes how the inscriptions and symbols on gravestones in Sweden increasingly reflect religious and cultural diversity. Moreover, the behaviour of mourners is increasingly eclectic. An individual family may select a sober traditional style for their child's grave but adorn it with personalised and softening touches, while putting their main energies into setting up a charity. The site where the ashes are interred may be minimally kept but a significant place visited regularly as a deliberate act of remembrance. Bradbury observed a huge range of behaviour at cemeteries, including for some people talking to the deceased person, but described them all as 'an intensely personal activity' (Bradbury, 2001, p 223). Walter (1996) describes the use of flowers in memorials and the range of floral customs currently prevailing across Europe, from the placing of a single flower with the body, to public displays of bouquets, sometimes on a mass scale, to mark the death of a public person, accident or disaster site, to artificial flowers in private roadside shrines and the tending of plantings on private graves.

As with funerals, memorials show a marked trend towards personalisation. Collier (2003) investigated the extent to which personalising trends had invaded tradition even in traditional social institutions such as military cemeteries. She provides examples from Japan, Russia and Israel as well as her own study in the US of how personal touches are introduced while retaining traditional structures. Everett (2000), in her research into roadside crosses in Texas, uncovered the practice of multiple sites, where families and friends of young accident victims had set up a 'memorial complex' in different places and forms. She describes, for example, how the family might set up the grave site, school friends put together an impromptu memorial using the contents of the young person's locker, while others who witnessed the scene of the accident erected a white cross. She also identifies the importance of the memorial placed at the accident site for the mourning of strangers who witnessed the accident but did not know the victim(s). And finally, in our tour of contemporary forms of memorialising, unsurprisingly, modern technology is enabling the development of new means and sites. Websites known as 'web cemeteries' exist to facilitate mourners posting and combining their personal memorials (Roberts, 2004), and in a contemporary take on war poetry, Searcey (2006) reports that soldiers in Iraq are using digital cameras and laptops to record the deaths of their friends. It remains to be seen the extent to which some of these personalised memorials survive in the way that traditional gravestones provide a permanent memorial. On the other hand, their relative impermanence in material terms is entirely commensurate with the age.

Seale discusses another interesting phenomenon of late modernity, in which 'the self may become a monument' (Seale, 1998, p 64) arguing that this is one way in which the western mind, tutored in the cult of the individual, bestows meaning on dying. Walter makes a similar point when he says that the authority of religion is replaced, in contemporary practices, with the authority of the self (Walter, 1994, p. 188). There is much about contemporary professional practice which encourages and possibly requires this behaviour of dying people. Young and Cullen (1996), from their study of terminally ill cancer patients in East London, pursue the notion that we desire 'a collective immortality' (Young and Cullen, 1996). They argue that there *is* continuity between the dead and the living and mechanisms which reinforce a sense of this continuity should be encouraged. This is an open understanding of the fact that life continues in the way it does partly because of the contribution made by those who have gone before, both individuals and passing generations or eras. The desire for a deceased relative or friend to be missed and remembered by a community is common among grieving persons. The 1662 *Book of Common Prayer* indeed expresses a common sense when it speaks of the 'community of all the saints'. Young and Cullen emphasise that death contains the potential to 'regenerate morality and human solidarity' by causing us to pause in the midst of life and reflect on the foundations for living. In this way, each individual death generates an ongoing monument.

Conclusion

We have seen in this chapter that the idea popularised in the 'modern death' thesis that advanced, secularised societies are devoid of ritual and symbolism to help them make sense of and deal with death, is no longer true. Contemporary societies demonstrate an increasingly complex set of procedures and behaviours as they negotiate the processes of commemorating, disposing and memorialising – as societies throughout history and across cultures have always done. When these new rituals do not turn out as expected, it causes great distress (as for Claire

Wallerstein [2006] who found the woodland burial site chosen by her father to be anything but idyllic and the process degenerating into dark farce). There are two marked developments which characterise this 'revival of death' – as Walter terms it. The first is the trend towards personalisation, the second an emphasis on affirming life in the face of death. Undoubtedly, there are some funerals which lack any investment with personal meaning and some lives which appear to 'pass away' without either commemoration or continuing memorial. Sometimes this is because of the particular category to which the person belonged or circumstances in which they died. Sometimes the particular circumstances of the death make it especially complicated to engage in social ritual. Sometimes mourners simply do not know what to do, or do not know how to achieve what would 'feel right'. Here we see another contemporary development. The funeral industry now includes within it a whole range of people, some frankly entrepreneurial, some seeing themselves as service professionals, who mediate between the old traditions and contemporary tastes and are arguably turning these individual personalised touches into new traditions.

Of what relevance is this detailed consideration of the events and procedures in the aftermath of the death for health and social care practitioners? First, nurses, doctors, social workers and the whole range of human service professionals need to recognise the importance for the present and future well-being of a bereaved person, of the way in which the practicalities of a significant death are handled, because they have enduring symbolic value. Second, they need to understand the symbolic processes which are woven through funerals and the pre- and post-funeral procedures and events, and to apply that understanding to the particular circumstances and context of individuals and their families. One issue which both social workers and clergy internationally have raised is the way in which the spiralling costs of funerals combined with rising public expectations about what is appropriate and desirable, are contributing to the further social exclusion of the most marginalised in our communities or leading to serious problems of debt (Carlisle, 1998; Drakeford, 1998; Bern-Klug et al, 1999; Adamolekun, 2001; Fox, 2005; Stoddart, 2006). Thus there is an important role for practitioners assisting families at the time of a death to help them clarify what is important for them, and why, and to help them secure the resources to achieve the funeral which is socially, emotionally and psychologically satisfying. Third, practitioners need to be alert to the needs of people who are excluded from attending the funeral or memorial service, whether because others deem it inappropriate (for example, excluding a learning disabled adult or child) or because they are physically unable to be there (for example, a frail or sick person, someone in prison). The impact of these processes being poorly managed was discussed in Chapter Four.

Key questions for practitioners

1. Am I working with someone who has lost a significant relationship and is planning, attending or has recently attended a funeral? What might they be feeling about the funeral (expectations, experiences, disappointments, comforting factors, good/bad memories)?
2. Does this person who is dying make reference to what they want to happen after their death? Have I given them the opportunity to talk about this? Can I support the family in planning together?
3. Am I working with someone who has lost a significant relationship and is excluded from/was not able to attend the funeral? What is the impact of this exclusion on them? Can/Should I intervene so that they can be involved? Can we create any alternatives to facilitate their mourning?
4. Is this person from a different social and cultural background to my own? What do I need to know/understand to relate to their needs in the immediate period after the death?
5. Are there cross-cultural or intergenerational conflicts or issues for this family? How can I help them to recognise and reconcile their different needs for ritual and ceremony?
6. Are there needs which I cannot address, and can I put them in touch with a more appropriate person?
7. Am I working with someone who has an unresolved experience of loss? What was their experience of the events in the immediate aftermath of the death? What memories of these events have stayed with them?

Notes

[1] At the time of writing there was a topical debate in the US as to whether members of the military who follow the pagan religion should be allowed to have pagan symbols on graves in the Arlington (Washington) cemetery.

[2] Although it should be noted that local laws regulate memorials, and church graveyards in particular may be quite restrictive about forms and wording.

EIGHT

Integrating theories and practices

Introduction

The approach of this book has been to examine the theoretical contributions from the different academic disciplines engaged in the study of death, dying and bereavement, and to set this alongside the professional context and issues faced by the different practitioners delivering health and social care. What is missing so far is any attempt to integrate these perspectives across disciplines and professions. The 'caring professions' have long but separate traditions of working with people who are dying or bereaved. Some, such as nursing and pastoral care, trace their whole tradition back to care of the sick and dying and are currently key members of the multidisciplinary palliative care team. Others, such as social work, found their niche in working with loss as they professionalised before Cicely Saunders, herself a one-time medical social worker, incorporated social work into her original vision of holistic care in the hospice. Psychotherapists from Freud onwards have dealt with the business of attachment and loss and the modern professions of psychiatry and clinical psychology continue to work with people who experience complicated grief. Psychiatry and psychology spawned the original formulations of grief counselling and grief therapy and continue to be active in its development, as Chapter Four explored. Clinical psychiatrists and psychologists tend to be less integrated into multidisciplinary palliative care teams, but in the forefront of dealing with suicide risk and post-traumatic stress disorder arising from disasters and other forms of traumatic loss.

Modern medicine has been rather more concerned with cure than care of the dying, but the development of palliative medicine as a specialism is spawning doctors who look outside of bio-medical models to address the wider needs of the dying person. At the same time, doctors are at the sharp end of the dilemmas created by their ever-increasing capacity to prolong life. This prolongation, such that we are increasingly dealing with a dying phase in which rehabilitation within palliative care is not only possible but desirable, has brought professions such as physiotherapists and occupational therapists into the frame, actively involved in helping the dying person to maintain optimal physical functioning in order that they can utilise this 'dying space' to address emotional and spiritual areas of their life.

The critique provided by the sociological analysis of modern death, combined with bereavement theories have had considerable influence on the work of these professions. There is now a general consensus among doctors and nurses that disclosure and openness are not only in the patient's best interests, most of the time, but their right. Social workers have focused on the empowerment of the dying person and the experiences of loss for both the dying and the bereaved, utilising their listening and 'low-key' counselling skills (Seden, 1999) alongside giving practical help on everyday matters. Chaplains have incorporated insights from psychology and counselling into their work, to the extent that a debate is ongoing as to whether pastoral theology has been lost in the process (Billings, 1992). However, this use of theory in practice represents a fraction of the rich theoretical resources available. It barely approaches a genuine interdisciplinary encounter, despite the rhetoric of 'holistic practice' which is repeatedly heard.

The context of late modernity

Four themes were discussed in Chapter One as the shapers of dying and bereavement in contemporary society. These themes have reasserted themselves at various points throughout this book. They have a direct impact on health and social care practice.

Causes and patterns of death

The majority dying of the twenty-first century in the developed world is that of older people, increasingly the 'oldest old', who become progressively frail and affected by one of the diseases or conditions of old age. This prolonged phase at the end of life has been brought about by improvements in general healthcare and advances in medical technology, both of which present policy makers, practitioners, individuals and families with socio-legal and ethical dilemmas. We have created a liminal phase before death, but the philosophical underpinnings, social rituals and policies for managing this phase have lagged behind.

Mrs Davies, aged 78 years, contacted Judy, a social worker on the care management team, about her daughter Megan. Judy had placed Megan, who has learning disability, in a supported living flat a few years previously. Megan had remained in daily contact with her mother and was emotionally and practically quite dependent. Gwen Davies had a chronic respiratory tract condition which was increasingly debilitating. She wanted Megan to be prepared for such time as she had to manage without her mother's support and, ultimately, her death. Judy soon realised, however, that Gwen also needed support for herself – practically, emotionally (she continued to have unresolved issues arising from her husband's death a few years previously) and in making her own preparations for death. Whilst Gwen clearly realised that she was in her 'dying phase', Judy had to fight to get the services Gwen needed to support her in daily living in order that her energies could be conserved for what to her was important business – such as returning to her place of birth in order to say goodbye. Without a terminal diagnosis and still presenting as relatively independent, Gwen was refused home care services. However, she continued to 'set her affairs in order', including arranging her own place in a nursing home when she could no longer manage at home, and died a few weeks after entering the home.

At the same time, some types of death, hitherto unknown or confined to the isolated few, are increasingly thrust into the public arena. The 'special deaths' of late modernity suggested in Chapter Four are particularly difficult for the bereaved to accommodate and stretch the helping resources of professionals, combining as they do trauma, stigma and existential challenge alongside the commonly experienced individual and social aspects of grief.

Simon's 19-year-old son died of a heroin overdose. Simon had no idea that he was a drug addict until the police arrived at his door to give him the news of his son's death. Simon had assumed the hours his son kept were down to his job as a chef in a city restaurant. A national newspaper and the local TV channel both featured the story, partly because Simon was a well-known local businessman, but also because of the details of the death – his son was found in a public toilet which was a well-known haunt of drug addicts. The shock, shame and anger against his son stayed with Simon; he found himself questioning the whole basis of his life. Eventually he joined a bereavement support group run by the Community Drugs Team, having felt unable to contact organisations such as CRUSE because the nature of his bereavement set him apart.

Globalisation of death

The opening up of death and dying through global issues and concerns may not appear to have immediate relevance for the front-line practitioner, but it has the potential to considerably enhance understanding and practice. One of the most interesting developments in recent years has been the establishment of the African Palliative Care Association, which has sought to rapidly translate best practice in western palliative care into culturally appropriate responses to the AIDS pandemic. In their engagement with international palliative care associations, these African colleagues have also contributed fresh perspectives. At various points in this book, the suggestion has been made that a transcultural approach, which seeks for common points of reference to aid understanding of difference, is an important refinement of multiculturalism. The global images of death that are transported around the world should serve to enrich our understanding and deepen our empathy.

Shifting boundaries between the public and the private

The shifting and permeable boundaries between what is deemed to be a private matter and what belongs to the public domain is one of the most striking aspects of death in late modernity. It runs through all the areas covered in this book. 'Private touches' in the public processes, events and places by which, and in which, people commemorate and memorialise their loved ones is an overriding trend and one which has particular application in therapeutic interventions. So, for example, the therapeutic benefits of ritual may be harnessed by recreating customised rituals and memorials with people with a learning disability, who were excluded from the funeral or had no opportunity to say goodbye. Social workers in specialist palliative care settings commonly undertake therapeutic groupwork with bereaved children, structured around activities which allow them symbolically to say goodbye and create their own memorials. Often a ceremonial element is included, such as lighting a candle. Nurses may assist parents of young children to create memory boxes, which the surviving parent may use to help children remember a relationship with the parent who has died, or to recreate a connection which they were too young to understand at the time.

Mike was 28 years old when diagnosed with an inoperable brain tumour. He and his girlfriend Katy had a new baby daughter. Mike was first admitted to the hospice for pain and symptom control. As his condition improved, Mike began to focus on his feelings about leaving his young family. At the suggestion of the social worker and with encouragement from his palliative care nurse, Mike and Katy began to create a memory box for their daughter. Sometimes they were absorbed in their intimate, private memories, at other times they insisted on sharing the contents of the box with Lisa, the nurse mainly involved in Mike's day-to-day care. It seemed important to Mike and Katy that others should acknowledge their family life. Mike also used these opportunities to share his feelings of loss that he would not see his daughter grow up.

Another significant development in palliative care which reflects this fusion of public and private is the objective of delivering professional standards of care in homely fashion, both through enabling people to stay at home while receiving specialist services and involving family members in their care, and through personalising and informalising professional care in institutional settings. It is extremely important that these aspects of service provision are understood in terms of what they symbolise, if they are to achieve the objective of best practice. Practitioners need to be sensitive to the tensions between public and private domains, including being prepared for the impact on themselves of moving out of the professional and into the private sphere. They also need to be aware of individual and cultural variations in the drawing of boundaries.

Sharon was a young mother with two small children who had cancer of the oesophagus. She was referred by her family doctor to a palliative care consultant for pain and symptom control but she was determined to continue to be treated at home. As she would not come to him, the consultant (Robert) visited her at home. He was unable to give her the best treatment at home because it required his close medical supervision. Seeing her at home, Robert felt exposed to the stress which her illness caused in the family, but Sharon seemed quite happy. She had accepted that she did not have long to live and wanted to spend us much time as possible with her children in their normal family environment.

The dissonance between public and private worlds in some stigmatised deaths is one of the most difficult aspects for the bereaved to deal with. The role of the media may be particularly instrumental in creating a sense of outrage, shame and deep ambivalence about the person who has died in this way, as well as exacerbating the shock of the death.

Julie's mother was murdered when she was sixteen. She had gone missing a few days previously, but the first Julie and her younger sisters knew of the discovery of her body was seeing it reported on the TV news. Because the body was found in a red-light district it was initially reported that her mother was a prostitute. Although it was later established that this was not the case, the media had by then lost interest in the story. Julie never really got over the experience of how the media portrayed her family.

Cultural pluralism

The ways in which death, dying and bereavement are marked and experienced are deeply embedded in cultural and religious tradition, shaped by cultural imperatives which, in turn, shape and indicate cultural change and identity. Health and social care in the societies of both the developed and developing world is delivered in contexts of cultural diversity, of individuals straddling cultures and of significant social transition. To provide an appropriate and culturally competent response in all situations is challenging and requires both knowledge and theoretical understanding. Robinson, a university chaplain, points out the importance of creating the opportunity for memorialisation for the student community when one of their number has died (Robinson, 2002). The following example accommodates cross-cultural perspectives.

Siu-Man was a Chinese law student, popular with his house- and course-mates and to all intents and purposes fully westernised. On a student night out he was killed in a road traffic accident. His friends were understandably shocked and distressed and began to plan their personal memorials, built around the activities which they had shared such as their five-a-side football team. The university contacted Siu-Man's parents and notified the chaplaincy. His friends had met his parents once and remembered that they did not speak a lot of English and seemed quite traditional Chinese. They also discovered in Siu-Man's room a shrine and remembered that he had said he was Buddhist. With the help of Chinese community leaders contacted by the chaplaincy, arrangements were put in place for a Buddhist ceremony and cremation, to take place soon after his parents arrived. Alongside this, a gathering was arranged at the university at which staff and students shared memories of Siu-Man and his friends brought along photos and played favourite music. His parents joined the occasion and seemed very touched. Some time later a tree was planted near the sports centre.

Applying theory to practice

Although the theories discussed in Chapters Three and Four have been extensively used in palliative care and bereavement training programmes, there has been surprisingly little research which looks at their use by health and social care practitioners in their work with dying and bereaved people. The exceptions to this are clinical psychologists and psychiatrists, who work within a clear theoretical orientation and approach. However, they work predominantly with bereaved people referred to them once a problematic grieving pattern has been established. If the extensive knowledge base about death, dying and bereavement is to assist us as individuals and societies in facing and accommodating these experiences, then it is important that it infuses the practice of a wide range of health and social care practitioners who might affect the path of the dying or bereaved person.

This book has suggested that greater integration of theoretical perspectives across the disciplines studying death could enhance our understanding. Table 8.1 provides an overview of the key elements in each discipline, set alongside each other so that their connections, but also distinctive contributions, can be seen.

Table 8.1: Typology of death – disciplinary focus

Psychology/psychiatry: concerned with loss/grief	Sociology/anthropology: concerned with death/dying	Philosophy/theology: concerned with death/dying
• Psychoanalytic/biological • Attachment/separation • Process of grief/relinquishing attachments • Continuing bonds • Intra-psychic focus	• Social construction of rite/ritual • Dying trajectory/ liminal state • Taking leave of dead/mourning • Memorialising dead • Societal/interpersonal focus	• Construction of life/ death • Construction of mortality/immortality • Taking leave of dead/ commending soul to God • Existential connection/ reuniting/resurrection • Existential/belief framework

In considering the application of these theories, it can be seen that psychological theories may help the practitioner understand the individual and their closest relationships; sociological approaches help to explain how what is going on around the individual and family shapes their personal experience; and contributions from existential thought suggest what might be helping or hindering the dying or bereaved person in making sense of it all, or, indeed, their need to find meaning at all. Parkes' model of bereavement as psychosocial transition integrates psychological and sociological dimensions of the individual experience. In Chapter Four it was suggested that an existential dimension could usefully be inserted into this model so as to more explicitly address the ontological and spiritual issues raised by bereavement (Figure 8.1). Broadening the notion of the existential search to the search for new or adapted models across all three dimensions, is helpful in understanding *how* individuals establish new assumptive models for their world. It is important to remember that while these searches may go on in parallel, they are experienced by the individual as a whole; if there is a crisis, it is brought about by the different challenges coming together, although one aspect may dominate. Using the evidence that crises of faith result in the re-establishment and strengthening of (reworked) original models as much as they result in the loss of faith, we can see that a reworking of the old models may lead to their re-establishment – for example, someone who sees themselves as needing an intimate relationship to function will find another partner. This psychosocial-existential model is also applicable to the process of dying – the dying person may reaffirm themselves as essentially the person they have always been, as much as others may revalue what is important.

Figure 8.1: Bereavement as psychosocial-existential transition

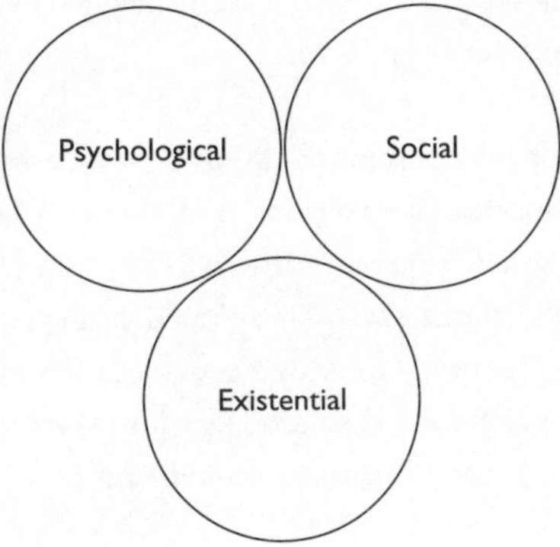

The following case study illustrates all three dimensions across the experiences of dying and bereavement in a complex family scenario.

> Mrs Baxter was referred to the community team attached to a hospice by the local social services care management team. The request was for bereavement support – Mrs Baxter appeared to be struggling with bringing up her teenage granddaughter, Laura, since her husband's death some two years previously. Laura was the child of their daughter, Susan, born when Susan was herself only 16. The family had had no contact with Susan for many years.

Mrs Baxter's health was poor and as she became more sick she was diagnosed as being in renal failure. She was offered a kidney transplant operation. She displayed great anxiety about this operation, being convinced that she would not survive it, even though it was explained to her that her condition without the transplant was life-threatening and that there were no particular complications. The social worker Carl said that, with hindsight, he wished he had listened more to her fears, since the extent of her agitation – for which there was no rational basis – probably indicated some deeper discomfort.

Mrs Baxter died of organ failure a day after the operation. In the middle of this crisis, as Carl was trying to offer emotional and practical support to Laura who was totally unprepared for this eventuality, Susan arrived on the scene. Laura had no recollection of her mother, but Susan explained that she had tried many times over the years to see her daughter but had been prevented by her own mother from visiting. Susan took Laura home with her. However, within a few days she contacted Carl, desperately wanting to talk about her feelings, and informing him that Laura had run away.

Carl began to work with Susan, who he recognised had experienced a very complicated double bereavement of both her parents (she had only just learned of the death of her father) as well as losing her daughter just when she thought she had regained her. Susan told a story of childhood abuse by her mother, with her father standing by and allowing it to happen. She had initially married Laura's father, but her mother opposed the relationship and it eventually broke down. After a series of abusive relationships, she met and married her second husband and has had a stable existence for over 10 years.

Carl engaged in a therapeutic relationship with Susan over a six-month period, during which Susan also had psychotic episodes. The initial focus of this work was the abuse she suffered as a child from her mother, including her anger towards her father for not protecting her. She displayed a high level of spiritual distress, talking of a punishing God and a God who seems not to care. Only when she was ready to draw a line under the memories of abuse, did she address her grief – for the parents and childhood which she wanted, and felt she had a right to. She then began to search for, and eventually to find, Laura.

At the heart of this situation is the attachment and separation problems experienced by Susan and Laura, leading to complicated grief in each case. There are multiple losses throughout the family history. Although we can see some resolution of Susan's grief, it is likely that Laura has a long way still to go as she reworks her perceptions of both her mother and grandmother. Laura's grief is also complicated by the fact that her grandmother's death was 'unanticipated quick' dying; she did not have a label of terminal illness and she was expected to make a full recovery from her operation. There are hints that the relationship was conflictual. These psychological problems are set into a social context in which there is likely to be little understanding of Susan's need to grieve – especially if the abuse was hidden – and the public roles and occasions around dealing with and marking the death of Mrs Baxter most probably fraught with tension and conflict between family members. Laura's response to the pressure of her situation results in her absenting herself from her grandmother's funeral. Although the background of family conflict is itself enough to cause Mrs Baxter's agitation as she approaches her operation, there seems to be a deeper level of distress in her fear of dying which does not respond to the standard psychosocial counselling approaches – often an indication of spiritual distress. Susan's crisis has a crisis of faith explicitly raised within it.

Translating theory into practice

Although the relevance of particular theories and concepts may be clear, their application in a way which influences how the practitioner works requires further translation. I suggest that four roles can be identified which cut across professional and disciplinary boundaries.

Creating a space for dying and grieving

Creating the physical, emotional, social and spiritual environment in which the dying or bereaved person may do their own preparation and deal with their own business is a role which different workers highlight as at the centre of their professional interventions and caring work. In part, this belongs to notions of the 'good death', the 'bad death' being one in which the control of symptoms is lacking, and circumstances allow no space or opportunity to prepare and to resolve troubling issues; fundamentally, the good death is a peaceful death in every sense.

Tim Roberts had developed a brain tumour at the age of 30. He was referred to Ella, an art therapist, following psychiatric inpatient treatment for severe depression. Tim had become very withdrawn when diagnosed and was resistant initially to engaging with the therapy, avoiding the topic of his illness altogether in the limited conversations which he had, including with his wife. The psychiatric episode appeared to have been triggered by existential despair – Tim had been brought up to believe that if he worked hard, the rewards would follow, and now he felt both cheated and a failure. When, after a month, Tim did start to draw, he became very anxious, angry and frustrated. Ella tried to create a calm accepting environment in which his drawings could be lodged. Gradually Tim started to communicate with his wife again. Tim presented Ella with his final drawing two days before he died (his previous drawings had been discarded). Ella believes that Tim had finally found a new way of valuing his life. He appeared to be reconciled with himself as well as with his wife.

The good death may not be a good or peaceful death as the workers would ideally see it. In the next example, the key worker, a hospice social worker, pushes the system to create the space in which a mother can fulfil her role as she wants, staying in control of her family life right up to her death.

Jackie was a 40-year-old widow who had breast cancer. Her husband had died in an accident five years previously following which her two young children had been referred for therapeutic intervention because of disruptive behaviour at school. Now in their teens, Jackie was fiercely protective of them and made every effort to keep social workers and other support services away. At times, this resulted in her failing to take advantage of treatments and support for herself – she attended the day hospice only once and often was out when home visits had been arranged. All the stops were pulled out for Jackie. When she was eventually admitted for hospice care her children were accommodated with her. Against all medical advice Jackie took her children on a last trip to London and their place in the hospice was held open for them to return to. For the most part Jackie remained hostile, defensive and ungrateful for the support provided, although she did begin to trust the social worker who arranged the family accommodation. The children also began to seek out other people to talk to about their fears. She died peacefully when her sister, whom she had asked to look after her children, arrived and took them out to the cinema.

An intervention used by many workers which has already been illustrated, is to assist in the creation of memories. Whilst observing that this is helpful to dying and bereaved people, workers are perhaps less conscious of the theoretical underpinnings of memorialisation and continuing bonds. Memories act as a trigger, which creates the motivation, the opportunity and the space for grieving to take place. Creating the accompanying rituals turns memories into remembrances and memorials. In other words, remembering becomes a socially sanctioned activity, whereas 'living through one's memories' attracts social disapproval. Thus, maintaining bonds, which many bereaved instinctively need to do, is allowed to have therapeutic potential. Chaplains tend towards a greater sense of the importance of ritualising memories, perhaps as a result of the personalising and customising trends which they have accommodated into the traditional funeral service. Kelly (2002) explores the role of listening and interpreting in co-constructing rituals for parents whose babies have died before or shortly after birth.

Assisting with the journey

Most people use this space to take further steps on their personal journey. Some are focused on the point they want to get to and others painfully make progress. The 'fellow traveller' is a familiar idea in pastoral theology and it involves four steps: *joining*, *listening*, *understanding* and *interpreting* (Lloyd, 1995). In different ways, some more consciously than others, the sensitive professional working with people who are dying or bereaved can be seen as 'getting in step' with the other person, perhaps helping them to see the direction in which they need to go, perhaps creating the conditions under which they take great strides, perhaps helping to accept a shortened journey.

Nicky was a young woman with breast cancer who was admitted to the hospice for the last few weeks of her life. She had a husband, Sam, and 3-year-old son, Liam. Cathy, a nurse on the bedded unit, admitted her and immediately felt they had a bond as women of a similar age with young children. Although Nicky and Sam were very positive in their attitude, actively looking ahead and planning for Liam's and Sam's future, they also had to deal with a lot of anger. They felt that Nicky's cancer had been misdiagnosed initially as mastitis and that maybe her death was needless or they could have had more time with better treatment early on. Nicky needed to confirm her identity as a mother, through planning for Liam's future, before allowing her grief at hers and their lost future together to come through. Cathy feels that by shouldering some of the burden and struggle for them, the palliative care team gave Sam and Nicky the space to complete these emotional and psychological tasks together. She describes Nicky as having embarked on her last journey when she entered the hospice, investing ordinary events with new meaning which seemed almost spiritual, although Cathy says she herself is not religious. Eventually it was Nicky who said that she had completed what she had set out to do and requested that a syringe driver be set up.

One way in which the worker can get in step with the other person is by assisting with *anticipatory grieving* before the death. Recognising when the relative or friend or the dying person themself is beginning to grieve, or needs permission to do so, requires awareness of the issues with which the other person is dealing and skill in picking up the clues that they are ready to engage with this aspect of their dying or bereavement. The grief may be for parts of the relationship already lost as well as anticipating life without the other person; it may be for lost expectations. In the example of Mrs Gwen Davies used earlier, it is in helping her daughter Megan to anticipate her mother's death that the social worker facilitates both Megan and her mother completing grieving for their husband and father. Megan is also assisted in moving on from being a dependent child.

Judy has been working with Megan to help her understand that her mum is getting more sick and will not be around forever. Megan refers back to her father's death and seems to be grieving for the loss of both parents. She needs reassurance that she will not be left to manage on her own and encouragement of her developing independence. Judy also works with the support staff on the network to assist them in helping Megan understand the implications of her mother's death for her and her future life. Freed from practical responsibilities, Gwen spends the time with Judy talking about her feelings of loss – the loss of her husband, which she has never got used to – and is looking forward, as she believes, to being reunited with him in heaven; the loss of her health and the freedom and independence that goes with it; the loss of her parenting role, although this brings with it a measure of relief and pride that she has done her job with Megan, and Megan is going to be OK. Judy also helps Gwen and Megan to plan the funeral with a local minister. Gwen is at peace and ready to die, and Megan, although initially very distressed when she realises that her mother will soon die, finds solace in this active engagement with her mother's death and is able to be with her when she dies.

Megan takes part in the funeral service, which Judy also attends, and 'receives' the mourners after, supported by her cousins.

Maintaining the spirit

Sustaining the person who is dying or in the throes of grief is at the heart of this work. 'Staying with the pain', 'just listening' and 'being there' are familiar roles to workers in this field. This implies workers giving of themselves as well as providing care. It is notable how many identify a personal connection, which enhances the support they are able to give to the other person. This willingness to 'stick in there' with the dying or bereaved person at their darkest moments is a crucial part of maintaining hope when otherwise helplessness might overwhelm.

Sarah, an occupational therapist working with Neil, who had motor neurone disease, discovered that they both had owned and ridden horses in the past and enjoyed sharing this interest. On one occasion Neil asked for help in loading photographs of his daughter, who also had motor neurone disease, onto his laptop and they sat together while his sadness overwhelmed him. Gillian, a care assistant on the day therapy unit also formed a connection with Neil. Gillian and Neil had both grown up in the same area at the same time and were able to share memories of people, places and events. Most especially, however, Gillian's daughter, who was the same age as Neil's daughter, had died about a year ago. Sometimes she just sat with him while he cried, where other people, she felt, avoided his pain. And she gave him his beer through a peg feed.

In this next example, acute spiritual distress threatens to destroy the peace of the dying person and her family.

Sandra was not known to the hospice when she was admitted from hospital. She was a woman in her 50s suffering from an inoperable brain tumour. By the time she was admitted she had already lost her sight. Maureen, the chaplain, was called in by the nurses because of Sandra's extreme agitation, screaming, calling out and making pronouncements of a religious nature – 'I'm going to burn in hell'. Her husband, who before his marriage to Sandra had been a church minister, seemed unable to communicate with his wife in her distress and in fact kept himself at a disatnce.

Maureen saw her role as trying to provide comfort for Sandra. She did not attempt to engage in spiritual ministry through conversation (and Sandra lost all speech in the end) but by gently holding and stroking Sandra's face, repeatedly assuring her that she was 'safe and secure'. This was the only thing which calmed Sandara, and the nurses, who had felt there was little they could do for Sandra, began to do the same. When Sandra died, a fortnight after her admission, she was peaceful.

Wounded healer

Sometimes the intervention is fraught with dilemma and discomfort. Some common feelings are experienced by workers in these situations, which arise at the personal–professional interface. Doctors share feelings of loneliness, vulnerability and helplessness with social workers, care assistants and chaplains; nurses and social workers are frustrated by the inadequacies of the system and also by service users who do not allow them to help; therapists find the intimacy of their contact opens up areas for which they were never trained and are challenged to push the boundaries; everyone is touched by the constant reminders of the darkness of suffering as they try to bring light into dying and bereavement. Sometimes the only healing which can be achieved is through death. This is perhaps particularly difficult for doctors to accept.

Lucy is a woman in her late 20s, married with two young children. Miriam, Lucy's GP, has known Lucy since the birth of her first child. Occasionally Lucy has mentioned how tired she feels but always coupling it with the stress of trying to manage a part-time job alongside bringing up her children – something with which Miriam can empathise. Suddenly Lucy presents with a serious swallowing problem. The endoscopy reveals that she has advanced cancer of the oesophagus. Lucy has researched her condition on the internet and believes that with the right treatment it is curable. She begins aggressive chemotherapy with Macmillan nurse support at home, but the tumour does not respond and it is concluded that her condition is inoperable. On a home visit, in which she encounters a lot of hostility from other members of Lucy's family (who believe that the diagnosis came too late), Miriam takes the decision to arrange admission to the hospice. Lucy is in the hospice for a few weeks before she dies. Lucy is saying that she does not want her children to come into the hospice and this limits Dave's opportunities to visit. Miriam visits Lucy a couple of times but she is uncommunicative. The nurses on the bedded unit and doctor caring for her at the hospice also find her disinclined to talk. Eventually, Lucy accepts that she is going to die and asks Dave to bring the girls to visit. She plans her funeral with the help of an older friend whose teenage daughter had died a couple of years earlier.

Miriam finds this case extremely difficult to cope with. On a personal level, she relates to Lucy as a young woman who should have had so much life ahead of her. She knows that she would have felt both sorrow and failure at leaving her children, but she is unable to connect with Lucy, even though they had always related very well before Lucy's illness. On the professional level, Miriam asks herself many times whether she missed the signs or mismanaged Lucy's treatment in the early stages, even though, rationally, she knows that she had organised the endoscopy as quickly as possible as soon as the indications were given to her and had got the best possible support available for Lucy while she was at home. She knows that she will feel a failure when she meets Dave and the girls again and privately hopes that they see one of her partners at the practice in the future. Miriam has found the whole episode very lonely, with the burden of expectation that as Lucy's doctor she should be able to cure her. At the end, Lucy's physical pain is controlled and she dies apparently 'peacefully'.

The model of the 'wounded healer', from pastoral theology, is perhaps the most helpful here (Nouwen, 1972). Very simply, it is out of shared weakness and vulnerability that the healer reaches out to heal. The model teaches us to value rather than avoid our own pain, perhaps from a similar personal experience, as the key element which enables the healer to connect and communicate with the dying or bereaved person.

Holistic approaches

Despite suggestions that the budget- and outcomes-driven priorities of health and social care have led to a fragmentation of separate tasks rather than a focus on the whole person, there are many arguments for suggesting that holism has been preserved in work with people who are dying and bereaved. A holistic approach is at the heart of the hospice mission; the social, psychological and spiritual dimensions of grief are recognised; doctors recognise the importance of psychosocial aspects in palliative care; nurses see spirituality as core; chaplains have become counsellors and only talk about religion if asked; social workers are rediscovering the importance of health issues; and therapists see the help they give with mobility as representing something both wider and deeper. Moreover, everyone subscribes to the view that the multidisciplinary team provides far better care than any individual profession could alone.

There is evidence, however, that this apparent consensus may hide a rather less coherent approach beneath the surface. First, the tensions between the different professional groups have never completely gone away in terms of hierarchies and roles, and even though the values underpinning our practice may be shared in specialist palliative care, the same cannot be said of all end-of-life care for older people. There are some suggestions that pressure to justify their role and cost-effectiveness is causing professions such as nursing, social work and chaplains to compete for aspects of care as belonging to their territory (Reese and Sontag, 2001). Nursing is beginning to raise its voice about the nurse's role in determining end-of-life care rather than merely carrying out the instructions, or monitoring the procedures, set up by doctors (Dobratz, 2005). The question of who should lead the multidisciplinary team in palliative and end-of-life care continues. For the most part, the clinical-medical model lead holds sway. It has been suggested that a needs-based model, with the lead given to the most appropriate professional as determined by the priority needs of the patient or family, would be more appropriate (Nyatanga, 2003). However, replacing one hierarchy with another does not fit with a holistic understanding of need. An approach which works to enhance understanding of the distinctiveness of each profession's contribution and how best to integrate those contributions, might better serve the pursuit of quality care.

I suggest that there is no one model for facilitating holistic understanding and practice in the individual caring encounter; in particular, our model should not be restricted to the tightly-knit multidisciplinary team. Leathard (1994) reminds us that interprofessional working has to operate through concepts and processes as well as through agencies. This may be through the organic development of relationships and understandings between professionals, or in a more organised fashion through collaboratory, cooperative or coordinated arrangements (Biggs, 1993). Ovretveit (1993) emphasises that whether the arrangement is a loosely coordinated network or an integrated interprofessional team, the key factor must be that all workers share a primary goal, grounded in meaningful user participation throughout all processes and at all levels. Holism should operate at the different levels of systems, communities, and individuals and families. Thus, our caring services need to be set up in such a way as to facilitate interprofessional and interagency communication, our assessment of needs and resources should incorporate the community and family, and our interaction with the person should be based on a whole-person approach. The end result might be that only one member of the multidisciplinary team is involved in a particular case, although this is likely to be unusual. However, that individual would be able to offer holistic care because they are informed by interdisciplinary perspectives, have available to them multi-agency resources, and are supported by the resources of their colleagues.

The following two case studies illustrate the opposite ends of this spectrum. In the first, a raft of services and workers are involved in community, day hospice and inpatient settings. The starting point for each worker is determined by their particular professional role and task, but their actual intervention reflects a holistic response to the needs expressed by the service users, resulting in a degree of overlap between them. In the second, a holistic response to the patient's needs is largely provided through one worker.

The Campbell family

Sarah, an occupational therapist (OT), first encountered the Campbells whilst working on a community team. She undertook an assessment of the needs of Karen Campbell, a young woman who had developed a particularly aggressive form of motor neuron disease. Sarah worked with Karen and her mother, Jane, on moving and handling techniques and safety in the home. During this time Karen's father, Neil, was also diagnosed as having motor neuron disease. Both Karen and Neil had care packages provided by the area care management team; one of Sarah's OT colleagues worked with Neil. Neil was in his mid-50s and his disease was less aggressive than the form which his daughter had.

From the beginning the family dynamics were very difficult. Jane found herself under great emotional and physical strain. She and Karen were very close as mother and daughter and as friends, having been in the habit of regularly shopping together and enjoying each other's company. As well as the practical issues, Sarah found herself providing emotional support for Jane, who confided in her about her feelings of loss concerning her daughter and her feelings of conflict between Karen's needs and those of Neil, her husband.

The family had moved into a small bungalow to make daily living easier, but the plan was for Karen to move into her own place. This was Karen's main goal, and although she already needed constant care, all the services worked together to achieve this end. A property and maximum support package was set up, but Karen never managed to move in. Her condition deteriorated very rapidly and she was admitted to the hospice where she died after a few weeks. By this time Sarah had moved jobs and was, herself, working in the hospice. Karen was not referred to her at this stage, there no longer being a role for occupational therapy.

However, Sarah did begin work with Neil, who was attending the Day Therapy Unit at the same hospice. Neil's speech was very impaired and their contact centred around helping him to get the most out of the communication aids, particularly his laptop. Through teaching him to use the technology, Sarah found herself getting to know Neil as a person and building a relationship with him. Using his laptop, Neil expressed his feelings of loss associated with his motor neurone disease, his frustration that his lack of physical mobility meant he could not even hug his wife when she needed comfort, nor could he articulate his love for his family. Gillian, the care assistant on the Day Therapy Unit formed a close bond with Neil. She seemed to be able to understand his speech better than other people and had significant shared experience. Neil talked to Gillian about what dying might entail for him and shared his deep sorrow, grief and guilt about his daughter's impending death. Other times Neil joined the relaxation groups and interacted informally with volunteers on the unit. He was visited by a befriender from the local Catholic church.

There were tensions between Neil and Jane and sometimes Neil talked about how he felt neglected by Jane in favour of Karen. Mostly, Gillian just listened but also tried to help Neil see how Jane must feel as a mother watching her child die and being helpless to do anything about it. Jane formed close relationships with the nurses looking after Karen and was also supported by the social workers, both before and after Karen's death. After Karen died, Jane was devastated by grief at the same time as she was also anticipating her husband's death. Gillian was able to empathise with the depth of Jane's feelings because of her own daughter, and Jane trusted her with these.

Neil was eventually admitted to hospital – there was no space on the hospice bedded unit when he needed it – where he died. Gillian and Sarah both felt disturbed that he may have died a lonely death, cared for by strangers. They attended his burial and were thanked by Jane for their support. She told them that Neil had told her he loved her just before he died and this was a great comfort to her.

The Campbells have between them a range of overlapping physical, social and emotional needs. The holistic care they receive is provided through a network of community services and hospice professionals and volunteers. There is no fully integrated care plan devised by a multidisciplinary team; rather, each worker opens themselves up to respond to the need presented to them, linked together in a loosely defined network of health and social care. Thus, with a background of community health, social care and housing services, the family, jointly and severally are supported through their shared experience of dying and bereavement. Neil does not receive counselling from the social workers but shares his grief with Sarah and Gillian in the course of receiving technical and physical support. Karen and Jane are a tight unit, but Jane finds support and a listening ear from the nurses caring for Karen. She is helped, by the social workers, to focus on her needs, to grieve before and after the deaths of her daughter and husband. Always there, is the skilled palliative care provided by doctors and nurses, which affords the dying space in which the family can focus on more than the physical aspects of dying. Perhaps most importantly, it is the care and support given to them as individuals, that enables Jane and Neil ultimately to be reconciled and mutually supportive of each other.

By contrast, in the next case, the patient has a close family and is directing her own course throughout with a high degree of independence. However, one worker, the physiotherapist, is particularly involved with her care. Although her role is technically limited to a specific physiotherapy intervention, through the provision of this service she offers emotional, psychological and social support which contributes significantly to the empowerment of the patient.

Marilyn

Janet qualified as a physiotherapist 30 years ago, but had worked in palliative care for only the last five years. This reflects the changes that have taken place in rehabilitation therapies and end-of-life care, with physiotherapy being offered as part of palliative care until the patient is too poorly to benefit. Marilyn was a woman in her early 50s with breast cancer and secondaries. She was very realistic about her prognosis but had one goal – to live long enough and be in control of her illness enough to organise and attend her daughter's wedding. Janet has a daughter the same age and felt she identified very closely with Marilyn. Marilyn was a very determined person who talked openly about her plans and the fact that she knew she was going to die. Janet found this quite difficult as it seemed to confront mortality head-on whereas her role is to bring about improvements in the person's functioning. However, Marilyn had great difficulties with breathlessness and this symptom alone caused her to panic and feel out of control.

Janet worked intensively with Marilyn helping her with breathing techniques in the Day Therapy Unit at the hospice over the 6-week period in the run-up to her daughter's wedding. She desperately wanted to help Marilyn achieve her goal and saw the breathing as 'central to the person Marilyn was'. She herself was pushed to the limits of her skills and challenged to try the newest techniques in order to help Marilyn. An intimacy developed between Janet and Marilyn through the nature of the contact – the use of touch, and the patient needing to trust the therapist in order to relax and benefit from the treatment. Marilyn was able to express her fears and sadness instead of being always positive and in control. Janet also obtained equipment and aids for Marilyn, including a state-of-the-art wheelchair which considerably improved her mobility inside and outside.

Shortly after her daughter's wedding Marilyn was admitted to the bedded unit having deteriorated rapidly. There was nothing more that Janet could do from a physiotherapy angle and the needs of other patients meant that she was only able to pop in once to see her before she died. She heard from colleagues that Marilyn had spent her last days planning her funeral and had made her own decision to turn off the oxygen. Janet knew that she had played an important part in Marilyn 'living until she died' and was sure that Marilyn was at peace when she died.

In conclusion – negotiating death

The concept of negotiation implies that one particular course of action or outcome is not predetermined and that participants may engage in a process to alter or determine that course to arrive at an agreed outcome or compromise. So how can death be negotiated, when it is quite simply the irrefutable outcome of existence? In answering that question we have to start with the fact that the knowledge of death is a fundamental feature of the human condition and the disciplines which study death have, in their various ways, addressed the implications of that. Second, the complexities of contemporary societies, including the health and social care needs and care systems within them, are having a significant impact on the experiences of dying and bereavement. This book has explored the changing patterns and contexts of dying, the new ways in which people are seeking to mark the passing from life to death, and the struggles which bereaved people experience in fluid and pluralistic environments in which traditional structures are disappearing or may seem irrelevant, yet new social and philosophical frameworks are sadly missing. In such circumstances, the fact of death may not change, but the manner of dying, the decisions and choices to be made along the way, and the implications for those who grieve are both shifting and negotiable.

Practitioners in health and social care cannot avoid death, dying, bereavement and loss, be they a palliative care consultant or chaplain in a remand prison. Negotiating the complex issues that arise in the situations in which death in the twenty-first century is played out, is a task that lies at the centre of contemporary health and social care. It is challenging and demanding of the individual practitioner, no less so because, sooner or later, our personal experiences and professional experiences overlap. This book has explored the many negotiations which must take place if the dying is to be personally acceptable and death to have social meaning. It is on the richness of the interdisciplinary encounter that we must draw as we seek to meet these challenges and to respond with knowledge, competence and sensitivity. A message left at the King's Cross site of the London bombings in July 2005 expresses its core: 'From another human being.'

References

Adamolekun, K. (2001) 'Survivors' motives for extravagant funerals among the Yorubas of Western Nigeria', *Death Studies*, vol 25, pp 609–19.

Adams, K. and Sanders, S. (2004) 'Alzheimer's caregiver differences in experience of loss, grief reactions and depressive symptoms across stage of disease', *Dementia*, vol 3, no 2, pp 195–210.

Addington-Hall, J. (1998) *Reaching Out: specialist palliative care for adults with non-malignant diseases*, London: National Council for Hospice and Specialist Care Services.

Addington-Hall, J. and Altman, D. (2000) 'Which terminally ill patients in the United Kingdom receive care from community specialist palliative care nurses?', *Journal of Advanced Nursing*, vol 32, no 4, pp 799–806.

Age Concern (2005) *Advance Statements, Advance Directives and Living Wills*, London: Age Concern England.

Ahmad, S. and O'Mahony, M. (2005) 'Where older people die: a retrospective population-based study', *Quarterly Journal of Medicine*, vol 98, pp 865–70.

Ahmed, N., Bestall, J.C., Ahmedzai, S.H. et al (2004) 'Systematic review of the problems and issues of accessing specialist palliative care by patients, carers and health and social care professionals', *Palliative Medicine*, vol 18, pp 525-42.

Ahronheim, J., Morrison, R., Baskin, S., Morris, J. and Meier, D. (1996) 'Treatment of the dying in the acute care hospital. Advanced dementia and metastatic cancer', *Archives of Internal Medicine*, vol 156, no 18, pp 2094–100.

Ainsworth-Smith, I. and Speck, P. (eds) (1982) *Letting go: Caring for the dying and bereaved*, London: SPCK.

Aitkenhead, D. (2005) 'The Things Left Unsaid', *The Guardian Weekend*, October 29, 19-27.

Allen, D. (2004) 'The right to a "good death"', *Nursing Older People*, vol 16, no 6, p 6.

Aries, P. (1974) *Western Attitudes Towards Death from the Middle Ages to the Present*, Baltimore, MD: John Hopkins University Press.

Aries, P. (1981) *The Hour of Our Death*, New York, NY, Knopf.

Arnason, A. and Hafsteinsson, S. (2003) 'The revival of death: expression, expertise and governmentality', *British Journal of Sociology*, vol 54, no 1, pp 43–62.

Arnold, E. (2004) 'Factors that influence consideration of hastening death among people with life-threatening illnesses', *Health and Social Work*, vol 29, no 1, pp 17–26.

Averill, J. (1968) 'Grief: Its Nature and Significance', *Psychological Bulletin*, vol 70, pp 721–48.

Barham, D. (2003) 'The last 48 hours of life: a case study of symptom control for a patient taking a Buddhist approach to dying', *International Journal of Palliative Nursing*, vol 9, no 6, pp 245–51.

BASW (1993) *People with a Terminal Illness – No Time to Wait*, Birmingham: BASW Trust.

Beckford, J. (1996) 'Postmodernity, high modernity, new modernity', in K. Flanagan and P. Jupp (eds) *Postmodernity, Sociology and Religion*, Basingstoke: Macmillan Press.

Ben-Amos, A. (2000) *Funerals, Politics and Memory in Modern France, 1789–1996*, Oxford: Oxford University Press.

Benbow, S. and Quinn, A. (1990) 'Grief, dying and dementia', *Palliative Medicine*, vol 4, pp 87–92.

Beresford, P., Adshead, L. and Croft, S. (2007) *Palliative Care, Social Work and Service Users: Making Life Possible*, London: Jessica Kingsley.

Bern-Klug, M., Ekerdt, D. and Wilkinson, D. (1999) 'What families know about funeral-related costs: implications for social work practice', *Health and Social Work*, vol 24, no 2, pp 128–37.

Biggs, S. (1993) 'Interprofessional collaboration: problems and prospects', in J. Ovretveit (ed) *Coordinating Community Care*, Buckingham: Open University Press, pp 186-200.

Billings, A. (1992) 'Pastors or Counsellors', *Contact*, vol 108, no 2, p 207.

BioCycle World (2006) 'Ecological funerals – potential industry in Sweden', July.

Bloch, M. and Parry, J. (1982) 'Introduction: death and the regeneration of life', in M. Bloch and J. Parry (eds) *Death and the regeneration of life*, Cambridge: Cambridge University Press, pp 1-44.

Boerner, K. and Heckhausen, J. (2003) 'To have and have not: adaptive bereavement transforming mental ties to the deceased', *Death Studies*, vol 27, pp 99–226.

Bonanno, G. (2001) 'Grief and emotion: a social-functional perspective', in M. Stroebe, R. Hansson, W. Stroebe and H. Schut (eds) *Handbook of Bereavement Research: Consequences, Coping and Care*, Washington, DC: American Psychological Association, pp 493–515.

Bonanno, G. (2004) 'Loss, trauma and human resilience: Have we underestimated the human capacity to thrive after extremely aversive events?' *American Psychologist*, vol 59, 20–8.

Bonanno, G., Keltner, D., Holen, A. and Horowitz, M. (1995) 'When avoiding unpleasant emotions may be not such a bad thing: Verbal-autonomic response dissociation and midlife conjugal bereavement', *Journal of Personality and Social Psychology*, vol 69, pp 975–89.

Boney, W. (1975) 'Care and concepts of hope: the resources of systematic theology', in R. Soulen (ed) *Care for the Dying*, Atlanta, GA: John Knox Press, pp 59–70.

Boros, L. (1973) *The Mystery of Death* (2nd edn), New York, NY: Herder and Herder.

Boss, P. (1999) *Ambiguous Loss: Learning to Live with Unresolved Grief*, Cambridge, MA: Harvard University Press.

Bowlby, J. (1969) *Attachment and Loss: Vol I: Attachment*, London: Hogarth Press.

Bowlby, J. (1973) *Attachment and Loss: Vol II: Separation: Anxiety and Anger*, London: Hogarth Press.

Bowlby, J. (1980) *Attachment and Loss: Vol III: Loss, Sadness and Depression*, London: Hogarth Press.

Bowling, A. (2003) 'Letter. Research on dying is scanty', *British Medical Journal*, vol 320, no 1205, pp 130–1.

Bradbury, M. (2000) 'Contemporary representations of "good" and "bad" death', in D. Dickenson, and M. Johnson (eds) *Death, Dying and Bereavement* (2nd edn), Sage Publications/Open University Press, pp 59-63.

Bradbury, M. (2001) 'Forget me not: memorialization in cemeteries and crematoria', in J. Hockey, J. Katz and N. Small (eds) *Grief, Mourning and Death Ritual*, Buckingham: Open University Press.

Brearley, J. (1995) *Counselling and Social Work*, Buckingham: Open University Press.

Brown, M. (2003) 'Hospice and the spatial paradoxes of terminal care, *Environment and Planning*, 35, pp 833–51.

Brown, P.L. (2005) 'Eco-friendly burial sites give a chance to be green forever', *New York Times*, 13 August.

Bruce, S. (1995) *Religion in Modern Britain*, Oxford: Oxford University Press.

Burton, A., Haley, W. and Small, B. (2006) 'Bereavement after caregiving or unexpected death', *Aging and Mental Health*, vol 10, no 3, pp 319–26.

Burton, R. (2004) 'Spiritual pain: origins, nature and management', *Contact*, 143, pp 3–13.

Bury, M. (1997) *Health and Illness in a Changing Society*, London: Routledge.

Butler, C. (2002) *Postmodernism: A very short introduction*, Oxford: Oxford University Press.

Caciola, N. (2000) 'Spirits seeking bodies: death, possession and communal memory in the Middle Ages', in B. Gordon and P. Marshall (eds) *The Place of the Dead; Death and Remembrance in Late Medieval and Early Modern Europe*, Cambridge: Cambridge University Press, pp 66–86.

Campbell, A. and Huxtable, R. (2003) 'The position statement and its commentators: consensus, compromise or confusion?', *Palliative Medicine*, vol 17, pp 180–83.

Campione, F. (2004) 'To die without speaking of death', *Mortality*, vol 9, no 4, pp 345–49.

Caplan, G. (1961) *An Approach to Community Mental Health*, London: Tavistock Publications.

Carlisle, D. (1998) 'The dying game', *Community Care*, 19 February, pp 16–17.

Cassidy, S. (1988) *Sharing the Darkness. The spirituality of caring*, London: Darton, Longman and Todd.

Catt, S., Blanchard, M., Addington-Hall, J., Zis, M., Blizard, R. and King, M. (2005) 'Older adults' attitudes to death, palliative treatment and hospice care', *Palliative Medicine*, vol 19, pp 402–10.

Challis, D., Darton, R. and Stewart, K. (1998) 'Linking community care and health care: a new role for secondary health care services', in D. Challis, R. Darton and K. Stewart (eds) *Community Care, Secondary Health Care and Care Management*, Aldershot: Ashgate.

Chan, C., Law, M. and Leung, P. (2000) 'An empowerment group for Chinese cancer patients in Hong Kong', in R. Fielding and C. Chan (eds) *Psychosocial Oncology and Palliative Care in Hong Kong*, Hong Kong: Hong Kong University Press.

Chan, D., Ong, B., Zhang, K., Li, R., Liu, J., Iedema, R. and Braithwaite, J. (2003) 'Hospitalisation, care plans and not for resuscitation orders in older people in the last year of life', *Age and Ageing*, vol 32, pp 445–9.

Chapman, A., Payne, S., Seymour, J. and Holloway, M. (2005) 'The Transition of Filial Piety to Parental Piety in End-of-Life Care', Paper to the 12th Hong Kong International Cancer Congress, Hong Kong University, Hong Kong, December 2005.

Charlton, B., Riley, J. and Best, S. (2005) 'Are both religious believers and atheists less depressed than the "existentially uncertain"?, *British Medical Journal*, Rapid response 26 August to Speck, P., Higginson, I. and Addington-Hall, J. (2004) 'Spiritual needs in health care', vol 329, pp 123-124.

Chong, A. and Fok, S.–Y. (2005) 'Attitudes towards euthanasia in Hong Kong – a comparison between physicians and the general public', *Death Studies*, vol 29, pp 29–54.

Christakis, N. (2003) 'The health impact of health care on families: a matched cohort study of hospice use by decedents and morality outcomes in surviving, widowed spouses', *Social Science and Medicine*, vol 57, no 3, pp 465–76.

Cicirelli, V. (2001) 'Personal meanings of death in older adults and young adults in relation to their fears of death', *Death Studies*, vol 25, pp 663–83.

Cicirelli, V. and MacLean, A. (2000) 'Hastening death: a comparison of two end-of-life decisions', *Death Studies*, vol 24, no 5, pp 401-19.

Clark, D. (2000) 'Death in Staithes', in D. Dickenson and M. Johnson (eds) *Death, Dying and Bereavement*, 2nd edn, London: Sage/Open University Press, pp 4–9.

Clark, D. and Seymour, J. (1999) *Reflections on Palliative Care*, Buckingham: Open University Press.

Clark, D., Dickinson, G., Lancaster, C., Noble, T., Ahmedai, S. and Philp, I. (2001) 'UK geriatricians' attitudes to active voluntary euthanasia and physician-assisted death', *Age and Ageing*, vol 30, pp 395–8.

Cobb, M. (2001) *The Dying Soul*, Buckingham: Open University Press.

Coleman, P.G., Ivani-Chalian, C. and Robinson, M. (2004) 'Religious attitudes among British older people: stability and change in a 20 year longitudinal study', *Ageing and Society*, vol 24, no 2, pp 167–88.

Collier, C. (2003) 'Tradition, modernity and postmodernity in symbolism of death', *The Sociological Quarterly*, vol 44, no 4, pp 727–49.

Collinson, P. (1990) 'The democratic solution', in R. Murles (ed) *From Patients to Customers: Are the NHS reforms working?* London:BMJ publications.

Collopy, B. (1978) 'Theology and the darkness of death', *Theological Studies*, vol 39, no 1, 22–54.

Connolly, M. (2003) 'Guest editorial. Time for non-cancer', *International Journal of Palliative Nursing*, vol 9, no 4, 40.

Cook, E. (2006) 'Saying goodbye our way', *The Guardian*, 19 August.

Costello, J. (2001) 'Nursing older dying patients: findings from an ethnographic study of death and dying in elderly care wards', *Journal of Advanced Nursing*, vol 35, no 1, 59–68.

Costello, J. (2006) 'Dying well: nurses' experiences of "good and bad" deaths in hospital', *Journal of Advanced Nursing*, vol 54, no 5, pp 594–601.

Coster, W. (2000) in B. Gordon and P. Marshall (eds) *The Place of the Dead; Death and Remembrance in Late Medieval and Early Modern Europe*, Cambridge: Cambridge University Press.

Coward, R. (2002) 'The problem with grieving', *The Guardian* (10 April).

Cowen, H. (1999) *Community Care, Ideology and Social Policy*, London: Prentice Hall.

Craib, I. (1994) *The Importance of Disappointment*, London: Routledge.

Crosby, C. (2004) Review of Felix, R. with Wilkins, R, 'The School of Dying Graces', in *Christianity Today* (December) 70.

Csikai, E. (1999) 'Hospital social workers' attitudes toward euthanasia and assisted suicide,' *Social Work Health Care*, vol 30, no 1, 51-73.

Cullen, L.T. (2006) *Remember Me. A lively tour of the new American way of death*, New York: HarperCollins.

Cumming, E. and Henry, W. (1961) *Growing Old. The Process of Disengagement*, New York: Basic Books.

Davies, C. (1996) 'Dirt, death, decay and dissolution: American denial and British avoidance', in G. Howarth and P. Jupp (eds) *Contemporary Issues in the Sociology of Death, Dying and Disposal*, Basingstoke: Macmillan.

Davies, D. and Guest, M. (1999) 'Disposal of cremated remains', *Pharos International*, vol 65, pp 26-30.

Davies, E. and Higginson, I. (eds) (2004) *Better Palliative Care for Older People*, Copenhagen: World Health Organization Europe.

Dawe, D. (1975) 'Drama on a barren stage', in R. Soulen (ed.) *Care for the Dying*, Atlanta: John Knox Press, pp 113–24.

Debate of the Age Health and Care Study Group (1999) *The Future of Health and Care of Older people: the best is yet to come*, London: Age Concern.

Decker, I. and Reed, P. (2005) 'Developmental and contextual correlates of elders' anticipated end-of-life treatment decisions', *Death Studies*, vol 29, no 9, pp 827–46.

De Bal, N., Casterle, B., Berghs, M. and Gastmans, C. (2005) 'Nurses' involvement in the care process for patients requesting euthanasia', *Nursing Ethics*, vol 12, no 1, pp 110–11.

Deeken, A. (2004) 'A nation in transition: bereavement in Japan', *Bereavement Care*, vol 23, no 3, pp 35–37.

Depaola, S., Griffin, M., Young, J. and Neimeyer, R. (2003) 'Death anxiety and attitudes toward the elderly among older adults: the role of gender and ethnicity', *Death Studies*, vol 27, pp 335–54.

Department of Health (1989a) *Caring for People: Community care in the next decade and beyond*, Cm 849, London: HMSO.

Department of Health (1989b) *Caring for Patients*, London: HMSO.

Department of Health (1998) *Modernising Social Services*, Cm 4169, London: The Stationery Office.

Department of Health (1999) *Reducing Health Inequalities: An action report. Our healthier nation*, London: HMSO.

Department of Health (2000) *The Expert Patient: A new approach to chronic disease management for the 21st century*, London: Department of Health.

Department of Health (2001) *National Service Framework for Older People*, London: Department of Health.

Department of Health (2002a) *Liberating the Talents*, London: Department of Health.

Department of Health (2002b) *Agenda for Change*, London: Department of Health

Department of Health (2004) *Independence, Well-being and Choice*, London: Department of Health.

Department of Health (2005) *Supporting People with Long-Term Conditions*, London: Department of Health.

Department of Health (2006) *Our Health, Our Care, Our Say*, London: Department of Health.

Dinh, A., Kemp, C. and Rasbridge, L. (2000) 'Vietnamese health beliefs and practices related to the end of life', *Journal of Hospice and Palliative Nursing*, vol 2, no 3, pp 111–17.

Dobratz, M. (2005) 'Gently into the light: a call for the critical analysis of end-of-life outcomes', *Advances in Nursing Science*, vol 28, no 2, pp 116–26.

Doka, K. (2001) (ed) *Disenfranchised Grief*, 3rd edn, New York: Lexington.

Doolan, E. and Brown, J. (2004) 'Lessons in death', *Nursing Standard*, Sept 15, vol 19, no 1, pp 22–3.

Dorff, E. (2005) 'End of life: Jewish perspectives', *The Lancet*, vol 366, pp 862–65.

Drakeford, M. (1998) 'Last rights? Funerals, poverty and social exclusion', *Journal of Social Policy*, vol 27, no 4, pp 507–24.

Edgar, A. (1996) 'The importance of death in shaping our understanding of life', in P. Badham and P. Ballard (eds), *Facing Death*, Cardiff: University of Wales Press.

Eisenbruch, M. (1984a) 'Cross-cultural aspects of bereavement 1: A conceptual framework for comparative analysis', *Culture, Medicine and Psychiatry*, vol 3, pp 283–309.

Eisenbruch, M. (1984b) 'Cross-cultural aspects of bereavement 2: ethnic and cultural variations in the development of bereavement practices', *Culture, Medicine and Psychiatry*, vol 4, pp 315–47.

Elder, N., Schneider, F., Zweig, S., Peters, P. and Ely, J. (1992) 'Community attitudes and knowledge about advance care directives', *American Board of Family Practice*, vol 5, pp 565–72.

Elias, N. (1985) *The Loneliness of the Dying*, Oxford: Basil Blackwell.

Elias, N. (1991) *The Society of Individuals*, Oxford: Blackwell.

Ellershaw, J., Foster, A., Murphy, D., Shea, T. and Overill, S. (1997) 'Developing an integrated care pathway for the dying patient', *European Journal of Palliative Care*, vol 4, no 6, pp 203–7.

Elwert, F. and Christakis, N. (2006) 'Widowhood and race', *American Sociological Review*, vol 71, pp 6–41.

Emke, I. (2002) 'Why the sad face? Secularization and the changing function of funerals in Newfoundland', *Mortality* vol 7, no 3, pp 269–84.

Engel, G. (1961) 'Is grief a disease?' *Psychosomatic Medicine*, vol 23, pp 18–22.

Environment Agency (2005) http://www.environment-agency.gov.uk/yourenv/consultations/902339. Funeral practices and the environment, draft policy.

Everett, H. (2000) 'Roadside crosses and memorial complexes in Texas', *Folklore*, 111, pp 91–118.

Exley, C. (2004) 'Review article: the sociology of dying, death and bereavement', *Sociology of Health and Illness*, vol 26, no 1, pp 110–22.

Feifel, H. (ed.) (1959) *The Meaning of Death*, New York, NY: McGraw-Hill.

Fetzer Institute (2003) *Request for proposals: End of life and the dying process: The role of spirituality/religiousness, human values and relationships*, Kalamazoo, MI: Fetzer Institute.

Feuerbach, L. (1957) *The Essence of Christianity*, New York, ET: Harper and Row.

Field, D. (1989) *Nursing the Dying*, London: Routledge.

Field, D. (2000) 'Older people's attitudes towards death in England', *Mortality*, vol 5, no 3, pp 277–97.

Field, D., Hockey, J. and Small, N. (eds) (1997) *Death, Gender and Ethnicity*, London: Routledge.

Field, N. (2006) 'Continuing bonds in adaptation to bereavement: introduction', *Death Studies*, vol 30, pp 709–14.

Field, N., Gao, B. and Paderno, L. (2005) 'Continuing bonds in bereavement: an attachment theory based perspective', *Death Studies*, vol 29, pp 277–99.

Finnis, J. (1995) 'A philosophical case against euthanasia', in J. Keown (ed.) *Euthanasia Examined: ethical, clinical and legal perspectives*, Cambridge: Cambridge University Press.

Firth, S. (1999) 'Spirituality and Age in British Hindus, Sikhs and Muslims', in A. Jewell (ed) *Spirituality and Ageing*, London: Jessica Kingsley Publishers, pp 158-174.

Firth, S. (2005) 'End-of-life: a Hindu view', *The Lancet*, vol 366, pp 682–86.

Fortner, B. and Neimeyer, R. (1999) 'Death anxiety in older adults: A quantitative review', *Death Studies*, vol 23, pp 387–411.

Foster, P. and Wilding, P. (2000) 'Whither Welfare Professionalism?' *Social Policy and Administration*, vol 34, no 2, pp 143–59.

Fox, P., Raina, P. and Jadad, A. (1999) 'Prevalence and treatment of pain in nursing homes', *Canadian Medical Association Journal*, vol 160, no 3, pp 29–33.

Fox, M. (2005) 'To die destitute today: what are the implications for social work?' *Australian Social Work*, vol 58, no 2, pp 188–98.

Franklin, L., Ternestedt, B. and Nordenfelt, L. (2006) 'Views on dignity of elderly nursing home residents', *Nursing Ethics*, vol 13, no 2, 130–46.

Frazer, E. (2000) 'Probably the most public occasion the world has ever known': "public" and "private" in press coverage of the death and funeral of Diana, Princess of Wales', *Journal of Political Ideologies*, vol 5, no 2, pp 201–23.

Fried, T., Pollack, D. and Tinetti, M. (1998) 'Factors associated with six-month mortality in recipients of community-based long-term care', *Journal of American Geriatric Society*, vol 46, pp 93–97.

Freud, S. (1917) 'Mourning and melancholia', in J. Strachey (ed.) *The Standard Edition of the Complete Works of Freud*, vol 14, London: Hogarth Press.

Frey, R. (2005) 'Intending and causing', *The Journal of Ethics*, vol 9, pp 465–74.

Fried, T., van Doorn, C., O'Leary, J., Tinetti, M. and Drickamer, M. (1999) 'Older persons' preferences for site of terminal care', *Annals of Internal Medicine*, 131, pp 109–12.

Froggatt, K. (1997) 'Rites of passage and the hospice culture', *Mortality*, vol 2, no 2, pp 123–36.

Froggatt, K. (2001) 'Life and death within English nursing homes: sequestration of transition?', *Ageing and Society*, vol 21, pp 319-332.

Gadberry, J. (2000) 'When is a funeral not a funeral?', *Illness, Crisis and Loss, vol* 8, no 2, pp 166–80.

Gamble, E., McDonald, P. and Lichstein, P. (1991) 'Knowledge, attitudes and behaviour of elderly persons regarding living wills', *Archives of Internal Medicine*, vol 151, pp 277–80.

Gardner, G. (2003) Letter 'Assisted suicide and euthanasia in Switzerland', *British Medical Journal*, vol 327, 52.

Gardner, K. (1998) 'Death, burial and bereavement amongst Bengali Muslims in Tower Hamlets, East London', *Journal of Ethnic and Migration Studies*, vol 24, no 3, pp 507–21.

Gatrad, A. and Sheikh, A. (2002) 'Palliative care for Muslims and issues before death', *International Journal of Palliative Nursing*, vol 8, no 11, pp 526–31.

Gatrad, R., Choudhury, P., Brown, E. and Sheikh, A. (2003) 'Palliative care for Hindus', *International Journal of Palliative Nursing*, vol 9, no 10, pp 442–8.

Georges, J.-J., Onwuteaka-Phlipsen, B., van der Wal, G., van der Heide, A. and van der Maas, P. (2005) 'Differences between terminally ill cancer patients who died after euthanasia had been performed and terminally ill cancer patients who did not request euthanasia', *Palliative Medicine*, vol 19, pp 578–86.

Gibson, M. (2006) *Order from Chaos* (3rd edn), Bristol: The Policy Press.

Giddens, A. (1991) *Modernity and Self Identity: Self and society in late modernity*, Cambridge: Polity Press.

Gill, S. and Fox, J. (2004) *The Dead Good Funerals Book*, Ulverston, Cumbria, Welfare State International.

Glaser, B. and Strauss, A. (1965) *Awareness of Dying*, Chicago, IL: Aldine Publishing Co.

Glaser, B. and Strauss, A. (1967) *Time for Dying*, Chicago, IL: Aldine Publishing Co.

Gonzalez-Ramos, G. 'The courage of caring' in C. Levine (ed), *Always on Call: When Illness turns Families into Caregivers*, New York: United Hospital Fund, pp 57–70.

Gordon, B. and Marshall, P. (2000) (eds) *The Place of the Dead; Death and Remembrance in Late Medieval and Early Modern Europe*, Cambridge: Cambridge University Press.

Gore, P. (2001) 'Funeral ritual past and present', in J. Hockey, J. Katz and N. Small (eds) *Grief, Mourning and Death Ritual*, Buckingham, Open University Press.

Gorer, G. (1965) *Death, Grief and Mourning in Contemporary Britain*, London: Cresset Press.

Gott, M., Seymour, J., Bellamy, G., Clark, D. and Ahmedzai, S. (2004) 'Older people's views about home as a place of care at the end of life', *Palliative Medicine*, 18, pp 460–7.

Grad, B. (1980) 'Healing and dying', *Journal of Pastoral Counselling*, vol 15, 50–4.

Grainger, R. (1998) *The Social Symbolism of Grief and Mourning*, London: Jessica Kingsley.

Grande, G., Addington-Hall, J. and Todd, C. (1998) 'Place of death and access to home care services. Are certain patient groups at a disadvantage?', *Social Science and Medicine*, vol 47, no 5, pp 565–79.

Grant, E. (2003) 'A Safari in Africa: Palliative care in cross-cultural perspective', *Contact*, no 141, pp 17–23.

Green, J. and Green, M. (1992) *Dealing with Death: Practices and Procedures*, London: Chapman and Hall.

Grogono, J. (2000) 'Letter. Sharing control in death: the role of an "amicus mortis"', *British Medical Journal*, vol 320, no 1205, pp 129–130.

Gunaratnam, Y. (1997) 'Culture is not enough: a critique of multiculturalism in palliative care', in D. Field, J. Hockey and N. Small (eds) *Death, Gender and Ethnicity*, London: Routledge, pp 166–86.

Gunaratnam, Y. (2001) 'Eating into multiculturalism: hospice staff and service users talk, "food", race, ethnicity and identities', *Critical Social Policy*, vol 21, no 3, pp 287–310.

Gunaratnam, Y., Bremmer, I., Pollock, C. and Weir, C. (1998) 'Antidiscrimination, emotions and professional practice', *European Journal of Palliative Care*, vol 5, no 4, pp 22–24.

Gushee, D. (2004) 'Killing with kindness', *Christianity Today* (December) p 62.

Guthrie, N. (2000) 'Praying for hope', *Christianity Today* (July) pp 46–8.

Guy, P. and Holloway, M. (2007) 'Drug-related Deaths and the "Special Deaths" of Late Modernity', *Sociology*, vol 41, no 1, pp 83-96.

Haak, N. (2004) 'Pilgrimages in partnering with palliative care', *Alzheimer's Care Quarterly*, vol 5, no 4, pp 300–12.

Haddow, A. (2000) 'Dying, death and after death', *The Journal of Religion and Psychical Research*, vol 23, no 3, pp 133–42.

Haley, W., Allen, R., Reynolds, S., Chen, H., Burton, A. and Gallagher-Thompson, D. (2002) 'Family issues in end-of-life decision making and end–of–life care', *American Behavioural Scientist*, vol 46, no 2, pp 284–98.

Hanley, E. (2004) 'The role of home care in palliative care services', *Care Management Journal*, vol 5, no 3, pp 151–56.

Hanson, A. (2006) 'Living with Gran, right to the end', *The Guardian* (14 October).

Hanson, M. (2006) *Living with Mother – Right to the Very End*, London: Virago Press.

Harding, R. (2006) 'Editorial. Palliative care: A basic human right', *id21 insights*, no 8 (February), pp 1–2.

Harding, R., Easterbrook, P., Higginson, I., Karus, D., Ravels, V. and Marconi, K. (2005) 'Access and equity in HIV/AIDS palliative care: a review of the evidence and responses', *Palliative Medicine*, vol 19, pp 251–8.

Hardy, A. (1979) *The Spiritual Nature of Man*, Oxford: Clarendon Press.

Harris, J. (1995) 'Euthanasia and the value of life', in J. Keown (ed) *Euthanasia Examined: Ethical, clinical and legal perspectives*, Cambridge: Cambridge University Press.

Harvath, T., Miller, L., Smith, K., Clark, L., Jackson, A. and Ganzini, L. (2006) 'Dilemmas encountered by hospice workers when patients wish to hasten death', *Journal of Hospice and Palliative Nursing*, vol 8, no 4, pp 200–9.

Hatzinikolaou, N. (2003) 'Prolonging life or hindering death? An orthodox perspective on death, dying and euthanasia', *Christian Bioethics*, vol 9, nos 2–3, pp 187–201.

HC Health committee report (2003–04) *Palliative Care*, London: The Stationery Office.

Heidegger, M. (1962) *Being and Time*, Oxford: Blackwell.

Hertz, E. (1907) 'A contribution to the study of the collective representation of death' in *Death and the Right Hand*, trs R. and C. Needham (1960), London: Cohen and West.

Heyse-Moore, L. (1996) 'On spiritual pain in the dying', *Mortality*, vol 1, no 3, pp 297–315.

Higginson, I., Astin, P. and Dolan, S. (1998) 'Where do cancer patients die?' *Palliative Medicine*, 12, pp 353–63.

Hinton, J. (1967), *Dying*, Harmondsworth: Penguin Books.

Hinton, J. (1980) 'Whom do dying patients tell?' *British Medical Journal*, vol 281, pp 1328–30.

HL Paper 21–1 of 1993–4, *Report of the House of Lords Select Committee on Medical Ethics*, London: HMSO.

Hockey, J. (1990) *Experiences of Death: An anthropological account*, Edinburgh: Edinburgh University Press.

Hockey, J. (2001) 'Changing death rituals', in J. Hockey, J. Katz and N. Small (eds) *Grief, Mourning and Death Ritual*, Buckingham: Open University Press, pp 185–211.

Hockey, J. and James, A. (1993) *Growing Up and Growing Old*, London: Sage.

Hoefler, J. (2000) 'Making decisions about tube feeding for severely demented patients at the end of life: clinical, legal, and ethical considerations', *Death Studies*, vol 24, no 3, pp 233–54.

Holloway, M. (2005) 'Care planning', in R. Adams, L. Dominelli and M. Payne (eds) *Social Work Futures: crossing boundaries, extending practice*, London: Palgrave.

Holloway, M. (2006a) 'Death the great leveller? Towards a transcultural spirituality of dying and bereavement', *Journal of Clinical Nursing, Special Issue Spirituality*, vol 15, no 7, pp 833–9.

Holloway, M. (2006b) 'Living with chronic illness: the example of Parkinson's disease', in P. Burke and J. Parker, *Social Work and Disadvantage: Addressing the Roots of Stigma Through Association*, London: Jessica Kingsley, pp 130–45.

Holloway, M. (2007) 'Spiritual need and the core business of social work', *British Journal of Social Work*, vol 37, no 2, pp 265–80.

Holloway, M., Chan, C., Chapman, A., Chow, A., Payne, S. and Seymour, J. (2005) 'What does it mean to die well? Beliefs and perceptions found amongst Chinese older people in the UK and Hong Kong', unpublished conference paper, Hong Kong International Cancer Congress, December.

Hopkinson, J., Hallett, C. and Luker, K. (2005) 'Everyday death: how do nurses cope with caring for dying people in hospital?', *International Journal of Nursing Studies*, 42:2, pp 125–33.

Howarth, G. (1996) *Last Rites: the work of the modern funeral director*, Amityville, New York, NY: Baywood.

Howarth, G. (1998) '"Just live for today". Living, caring, ageing and dying', *Ageing and Society*, vol 18, pp 673–89.

Howell, D. (2004) 'Guest editorial. Integrated care: hospice and palliative care services lead the way', *International Journal of Palliative Nursing*, vol 10, no 4, p 60.

Howse, K. (2004) 'Religion and spirituality in later life', *Generations Review*, vol 14, no 4, pp 6–19.

Hsu, M.-T., Kahn, D., Yee, D.-H. and Lee, W.-L. (2004) 'Recovery through reconnection: a cultural design for family bereavement in Taiwan', *Death Studies*, vol 28, pp 761–86.

Huang, Z. and Ahronheim, J. (2000) 'Nutrition and hydration in terminally ill patients: an update', *Clinics in Geriatric Medicine*, vol 16, no 2, pp 313-25.

Hudson, B. (2000) 'Inter-agency collaboration – a sceptical view', in A. Brechin, H. Brown and M. Eby (eds) *Critical Practice in Health and Social Care*, London: Sage/Open University, pp 253–74.

Hurst, S. and Mauron, A. (2006) 'The ethics of palliative care and euthanasia: exploring common values', *Palliative Medicine*, vol 20, 107–12.

Huxtable, R. (2004) 'Get out of jail free? The doctrine of double effect in English law', *Palliative Medicine*, vol 18, pp 62–68.

IOM (Institute of Medicine) (2001) *Crossing the Quality Chasm: A New Health System for the 21st Century*, Washington: National Academies of Sciences.

IOM (2003) *Describing Death in America: what we need to know*, Washington: National Academies of Sciences.

Irish, D. (ed.) (1993), *Ethnic Variations in Dying, Death and Grief*, London: Taylor & Francis.

Jacobs, S., Mazure, C. and Prigerson, H. (2000) 'Diagnostic criteria for traumatic grief', *Death Studies*, vol 24, pp 185–99.

Jack, C., Jones, L., Jack, B., Gambles, M, Murphy, D. and Ellerenshaw, J. (2004) 'Research letters. Towards a good death: the impact of the care of the dying pathway in an acute stroke unit', *Age and Ageing*, vol 33, no 6, pp 625–26.

Jack, C., Jones, L., Jack, B., Gambles, M, Murphy, D. and Ellerenshaw, J. (2005) 'Reply to Shah, S. 'The Liverpool Care Pathway: its impact on improving the care of the dying', *Age and Ageing*, vol 34, no 1, pp 197-8.

Jackson, E. (1982) *Counselling the Dying*, London: SCM Press.

James, A. and Wells, A. (2002) 'Death beliefs, superstitious beliefs and health anxiety', *British Journal of Clinical Psychology*, vol 41, pp 43–53.

Jaspers, K. (1967) *Philosophical Faith and Revelation*, London: Collins.

Jecker, N. and Schneiderman, L. (1994) 'Is dying young worse than dying old?', *The Gerontologist*, vol 34, pp 66–72.

Jenkins, R. (2004) *Social Identity* (2nd edn), London: Routledge.

Jewell, A. (1999) (ed.) *Spirituality and Ageing*, London: Jessica Kingsley.

Johansen, S., Helen, J., Kaasa, S., Loge, J. and Materstvedt, L. (2005) 'Attitudes towards, and wishes for, euthanasia in advanced cancer patients at a palliative medicine unit', *Palliative Medicine*, vol 19, pp 454–60.

Johnson, C. and Barer, B. (1997) *Life beyond 85 years: The aura of survivorship*, New York, NY: Springer.

Johnson, M., Cullen, L., Heatley, R. and Hockey, J. (2001) *The Psychology of Death: An exploration of the impact of bereavement on the purchasers of 'at need' funerals*, Bristol: International Institute on Health and Ageing, University of Bristol.

Jones, J. and Willis, D. (2003) 'Letter. What is a good death?', *British Medical Journal*, vol 327, no 7408, pp 224.

Jonker, G. (1997) 'Death, gender and memory: remembering loss and burial as a migrant', in D. Field, J. Hockey and N. Small (eds) *Death, Gender and Ethnicity*, London: Routledge, pp 187–201.

Jung, C. (1959) 'The soul and death', in H. Feifel (ed) *The Meaning of Death*, New York, NY: McGraw-Hill.

Jungel, E. (1975) *Death, the Riddle and the Mystery*, Edinburgh: Saint Andrew Press.

Kalbag, R. (2003) 'Letter. Do we really know what happens in this country?', *British Medical Journal*, vol 327, no 7408, pp 226.

Kellaher, L., Prendergast, D. and Hockey, J. (2005) 'In the shadow of the traditional grave', *Mortality*, vol 10, no 4, pp 237–50.

Kellehear, A. (1984) 'Are we a death-denying society? A sociological review', *Social Science and Medicine*, vol 18, no 9, pp 713–21.

Kellehear, A. (1984) 'The sociology of death and dying: an overview', *Australian Social Work*, vol 37, nos 3 and 4, pp 3–9.

Kellehear, A. (1990) *Dying of Cancer. The Final Year of Life*, London: Harwood Academic.

Kellehear, A. (2000) 'Spirituality and palliative care: a model of needs', *Palliative Medicine*, vol 14, pp 149–55.

Kelly, E. (2002) *Marking Life and Death: Co-constructing welcoming and funeral rituals for babies dying in utero or shortly after birth*, Contact Pastoral Monograph, no 12, Edinburgh: Contact Pastoral Trust.

Kikule, E. (2003) 'A good death in Uganda; a survey of needs for palliative care for terminally ill people in urban areas', *British Medical Journal*, vol 327, no 7408, pp 192–4.

Kissane, M. and McLaren, S. (2006) 'Sense of belonging as predictor of reasons for living in older adults', *Death Studies*, vol 30, no 3, pp 243–58.

Klass, D. (1988) *Parental Grief: Solace and Resolution*, New York, NY: Springer.

Klass, D. (2006) 'Continuing conversation about continuing bonds', *Death Studies*, vol 30, pp 843–58.

Klass, D. and Goss, R. (1999) 'Spiritual bonds to the dead in cross-cultural and historical perspective: comparative religion and modern grief', *Death Studies*, vol 23, no 6, pp 547–67.

Klass, D., Silverman, P. and Nickman, S. (eds) (1996) *Continuing Bonds: New understandings of grief*, London: Taylor & Francis.

Klinkenberg, M., Visser, G., Van Groenou, M., Van der Wal, G., Deeg, D. and Willems, D. (2005) 'The last 3 months of life: care, transitions and the place of death of older people', *Health and Social Care in the Community*, vol 13, no 5, pp 420–30.

Koenig, H.G., George, L.K. and Peterson, B.L. (1998) 'Religiosity and remission of depression in medically ill older patients', *American Journal of Psychiatry*, vol 155, no 4, pp 536–42.

Komaromy, C. (2000) 'The sight and sound of death: the management of dead bodies in residential and nursing homes', *Mortality*, vol 5, no 3, pp 299–315.

Komaromy, C. and Hockey, J. (2001) '"Naturalising" death among older adults in residential care', in J. Hockey, J. Katz and N. Small (eds) *Grief, Mourning and Death Ritual*, Buckingham: Open University Press.

Kristjanson, L. and Christakis, N. (2005) 'Editorial. Investigating euthanasia: methodological, ethical and clinical considerations', *Palliative Medicine*, vol 19, pp 575–7.

Kubler-Ross, E. (1970) *On Death and Dying*, London: Tavistock Publications Ltd.

Kubler-Ross, E. (1975) *Death: The final stage of growth*, Englewood Cliffs, NJ: Prentice Hall.

Kung, H. (1984) *Eternal Life?*, London: Collins.

Laderman, G. (2003) *Rest in Peace: A cultural history of death and the funeral home in twentieth-century America*, Oxford: Oxford University Press.

Larson, J., Franzen-Dahlin, A., Billing, E., Murray, V. and Wredling, R. (2005) 'Spouse's life situation after partner's stroke event: psychometric testing of a questionnaire', *Methodological Issues in Nursing Research*, vol 52, no 3, pp 300–6.

Lawton, J. (2000) *The Dying Process: Patients' Experiences of Palliative Care*, London: Routledge.

Leathard, A. (1994) ;Interprofessional developments in Britain: an overview', in A. Leathard (ed) *Going Inter-Professional*, London: Routledge, pp 3-37.

Leese, B., Din, I., Darr, A., Walker, R., Heywood, P. and Allgar, V. (2004) '*Early Days Yet'. Evaluation of the Primary Care Cancer Lead Clinician (PCCL) Initiative*, University of Leeds: Centre for Research in Primary Care/London: Department of Health.

Leichtentritt, R. (2002) 'Euthanasia: Israeli Social Workers' Experiences, Attitudes and Meanings', *British Journal of Social Work*, vol 32, no 4, pp 397–413.

Leland, J. (2006) 'It's my funeral and I'll serve ice cream if I want to', *The New York Times* (20 July).

Lewis, C.S. (1966) *A Grief Observed*, London: Faber & Faber.

Lewis, J. and Glennerster, H. (1996) *Implementing the New Community Care*, Buckingham: Open University Press.

Lewis, J., Bernstock, P., Bovell, V. and Wookey, F. (1997) 'Implementing care management: issues in relation to the new community care', *British Journal of Social Work*, vol 27, no 1, pp 5–24.

Lewis, M. and Trzinski, A. (2006) 'Counselling older adults with dementia who are dealing with death: innovative interventions for practitioners', *Death Studies*, vol 30, pp 777–87.

Lifton, R. (1979) *The Broken Connection*, New York, NY: Simon & Schuster.

Lindemann, E. (1944) 'Symptomatology and management of acute grief', *American Journal of Psychiatry*, vol 101, pp 141–49.

Lindemann, E. (1976) 'Grief and grief management', *Journal of Pastoral Care*, vol 30, pp 198–200.

Linnane, B. (2001) 'Dying with Christ: Rahner's Ethics of Discipleship', *The Journal of Religion*, vol 81, no 2, pp 228–48.

Littlewood, J. (1992) *Aspects of Grief: Bereavement in adult life*, London: Routledge.

Lloyd, M. [M. Holloway] (1992) 'Tools for many trades: reaffirming the use of grief counselling by health, welfare and pastoral workers', *British Journal of Guidance and Counselling*, vol 20, no 2, pp 151–64.

Lloyd, M. [M. Holloway] (1995) *Embracing the Paradox: Pastoral care with dying and bereaved people*, Contact Pastoral Monographs No 5, Edinburgh: Contact Pastoral Limited Trust.

Lloyd, M. [M. Holloway] (1996) 'Philosophy and religion in the face of death and bereavement', *Journal of Religion and Health*, vol 35, no 4, pp 295–310.

Lloyd, M. [M. Holloway] (1997) 'Dying and bereavement, spirituality and social work in a market economy of welfare', *British Journal of Social Work*, vol 27, no 2, pp 175–90.

Lloyd, M. [M. Holloway] (2000) 'Where has all the care management gone? The challenge of Parkinson's disease to the health and social care interface', *British Journal of Social Work*, vol 30, no 6, pp 737–54.

Lloyd, M. [M. Holloway] (2002a) 'Care management', in R. Adams, L. Dominelli and M. Payne (eds) *Critical Practice in Social Work*, London: Palgrave, pp 159–68.

Lloyd, M. [M. Holloway] (2002b) 'A framework for working with loss', in N. Thompson (ed.) *Loss and Grief: A guide for human services practitioners*, London: Palgrave, pp 208–20.

Lockhart, L., Ditto, P., Danks, J., Coppola, K. and Smucker, W. (2001) 'The stability of older adults' judgments of fates better and worse than death', *Death Studies*, vol 25, pp 299–317.

Lorenz, K., Asch, S., Rosenfield, K., Liu, H. and Ettner, S. (2004) 'Hospice admission practices: where does hospice fit in the continuum of care?' *Journal of the American Geriatrics Society*, vol 52, pp 725–30.

Low, J. and Payne, S. (1996) 'The "good" and "bad death" perceptions of health professionals working in palliative care', *European Journal of Cancer Care*, 5, pp 237–41.

Loyalka, M.D. (2005) 'Putting the Fun in Funerals', *Business Week Online* (17 November).

Lund, D. (ed) (1989a) *Older Bereaved Spouses: Research with practical applications*, New York, NY: Hemisphere Publishing.

Lund, D. (1989b) 'Conclusions about bereavement in later life and implications for interventions and future research', in D. Lund (ed.) (1989) *Older Bereaved Spouses: Research with practical applications*, New York, NY: Hemisphere Publishing, pp 217–31.

Luptak, M. (2004) 'Social work and end-of-life care for older people: a historical perspective', *Health and Social Work*, vol 29, no 1, pp 7–15.

Lymbery, M. (1998) 'Care management and professional autonomy: The impact of community care legislation on social work with older people', *British Journal of Social Work*, vol 28, no 6, pp 863–78.

Lynn, J., Teno, J.M., Phillips, R.S., Wu, A.W., Desbiens, N., Harrold, J., Claessens, M.T., Wenger, N., Kreling, B. and Connors Jr., A.F. (1997) 'Perceptions by family members of the dying experience of older and seriously ill patients', *Annals of Internal Medicine*, 126, pp 97–106.

Mackay, M. (1993) *Dementia and Bereavement*, Stirling: Dementia Services Development Centre, University of Stirling.

Mackelprang, R.W. and Mackelprang, R.D. (2005) 'Historical and contemporary issues in end-of-life decisions: implications for social work', *Social Work*, vol 50, no 4, pp 315–24.

MacKinlay, E. (2001) *The Spiritual Dimension of Ageing*, London: Jessica Kingsley.

Macquarrie, J. (1973) *An Existentialist Theology*, London: SCM Press.

Macquarrie, J. (1982) *In Search of Humanity*, London: SCM Press.

Mak, J. and Clinton, M. (1999) 'Promoting a good death: an agenda for outcomes research – a review of the literature', *Nursing Ethics*, vol 6, no 2, pp 97–106.

Mak, Y. and Elwyn, G. (2005) 'Voices of the terminally ill: uncovering the meaning of desire for euthanasia', *Palliative Medicine*, vol 19, pp 343–50.

Malkinson, R., Rubin, S. and Witztum, E. (2006) 'Therapeutic issues and the relationship to the deceased: working clinically with the two-track model of bereavement', *Death Studies*, vol 30, pp 797–815.

Manning, D. (2001) *The Funeral. A chance to touch, a chance to serve, a chance to heal*, Oklahoma City, OK: In-Sight Books.

Marris, P. (1974) *Loss and Change*, London: Routledge and Kegan Paul.

Martineau, I., Blondeau, D. and Godin, G. (2003) 'Choosing a place of death: the influence of pain and of attitude toward death', *Journal of Applied Social Psychology*, vol 33, no 9, pp 1973–93.

Martin-Matthews, A. (1999) 'Widowhood: dominant renditions, changing demography, and variable meaning', in S. Neysmith (ed.) *Critical Issues for Future Social Work Practice with Aging Persons*, New York: Columbia University Press.

Marwit, S. and Meuser, T. (2005) 'Development of a short form inventory to assess grief in caregivers of dementia patients', *Death Studies*, vol 29, pp 191–205.

Materstvedt, L., Clark, D., Ellershaw, J., Forde, R., Gravgaard, A.-M., Muller-Busch, H., Sales, J. and Raplin, C.-H. (2003) 'Euthanasia and physician-assisted suicide: a view from an EAPC Ethics Task Force', *Palliative Medicine*, vol 17, pp 97–101.

Matthews, L. and Marwit, S. (2004) 'Complicated grief and the trend toward cognitive-behavioral therapy', *Death Studies*, vol 28, pp 849–63.

Matthews, S. (1986) *Friendship through the life course: oral biographies in old age*, London: Sage.

Maudlin, M. (2001) '"Dying together". Review of D. Hallock, "Six months to live: learning from a young man with cancer"', in *Christianity Today* (3 September) 106–7.

Maughan, G. (1988) *The Observer* (27 March).

McBride, J. and Armstrong, G. (1995) 'The spiritual dynamics of post-traumatic stress disorder', *Journal of Religion and Health*, vol 34, no 1, 5–16.

McCalman, J.A. (1990) *The Forgotten People: Carers in three minority ethnic communities in Southwark*, London: King's Fund.

McClain, C., Rosenfield, B. and Breitbart, W. (2003) 'Effect of spiritual well-being on end-of-life despair in terminally-ill cancer patients', *The Lancet*, vol 361, pp 1603–7.

McGrath, P. (2003) 'Religiosity and the challenge of terminal illness', *Death Studies*, vol 27, pp 881–99.

McNamara, B. (2001) *Fragile Lives: Death, Dying and Care*, Buckingham: Open University Press.

McNamara, B., Waddell, C. and Colvin, M. (1994) 'The institutionalization of the good death', *Social Science and Medicine*, vol 39, no 11, pp 1501–8.

McSherry, W. (2007) *Making Sense of Spirituality in Nursing Practice: An Integrated Approach*, 2nd edn, London: Harcourt Publishers.

Means, R. and Smith, R. (1998) *Community Care: Policy and Practice* (2nd edn), London: Macmillan.

Meilaender, G. (2005) 'Living life's end', *First Things: A Monthly Journal of Religion & Public Life*, Issue 153, pp 17–21.

Metcalfe, P. and Huntington, R. (1991) *Celebrations of Death. The anthropology of mortuary ritual* (2nd edn) Cambridge: Cambridge University Press.

Midwinter, E. (1987) *Redefining Old Age*, London: Centre for Policy on Ageing.

Miller, S. and Ryndes, T. (2005) 'Quality of life at the end of life: the public health perspective, *Generations*, vol 29, no 2, pp 41–7.

Milligan, C. (2000) 'Bearing the burden: towards a restructured geography of caring', *Area*, 32, 49–58.

Mitchell, G. and Seamark, D. (2003) 'Dying in the community: general practitioner treatment of community-based patients analysed by chart audit', *Palliative Medicine*, vol 17, pp 289–92.

Mitford, J. (1963) *The American Way of Death*, 1st edn, London: Hutchinson.

Mitford, J. (2000) *The American Way of Death Revisited*, New York, NY: Vintage Books.

Mohrmann, M. (2006) 'Whose interests are they anyway?', *Journal of Religious Ethics*, vol 34, no 1, pp 141–50.

Moltman, J. (1989) *Creating a Just Future: The politics of peace and the ethics of creation in a threatened world*, London: SCM Press.

Moore, P.J., and Phillips, L. (1994) 'Black American communities: Coping with death', in Dane and Levine (eds), *AIDS and the new orphans: coping with death*, Westport, CT: Greenwood Publishing.

Morgan, J. (1995) 'Living our dying and grieving: historical and cultural attitudes', in H. Wass and R. Neimeyer (eds) *Dying: Facing the facts* (3rd edn), Washington DC: Taylor & Francis.

Morita, T., Miyashita, M., Kimura, R., Adachi, I. and Shima, Y. (2004) 'Emotional burden of nurses in palliative sedation therapy', *Palliative Medicine*, vol 18, pp 550–7.

Moss, B. (2005) *Religion and Spirituality*, Lyme Regis: Russell House Publishing.

Moss, M. and Moss, S. (1989) 'Death of the very old', in K. Doka (ed.) *Disenfranchised Grief: Recognising hidden sorrow*, Lexington, MA: Lexington Books, pp 213–27.

NCHSPCS (National Council for Hospices and Specialist Palliative Care Services) (1995) *Opening Doors: Improving access to hospital and specialist palliative care services by members of the black and ethnic minority communities*, London: NCHSPCS.

NCHSPCS (2001) *Wider Horizons*, London: NCHSPCS.

National Funeral Directors Association, www.nfda.org, accessed 22 September 2006.

Neimeyer, R. (ed.) (2001) *Meaning Reconstruction and the Experience of Loss*, Washington, DC: American Psychological Association.

Neimeyer, R. and Anderson, A. (2002) 'Meaning reconstruction theory', in N. Thompson (ed.) *Loss and Grief. A guide for human services practitioners*, London: Palgrave.

Neimeyer, R., Baldwin, S. and Gillies, J. (2006) 'Continuing bonds and reconstructing meaning: mitigating complications in bereavement', *Death Studies*, vol 30, pp 715–38.

Neimeyer, R., Prigerson, H. and Davies, B. (2002) 'Mourning and memory', *American Behavioral Scientist*, vol 26, no 2, pp 235–51.

Neimeyer, R., Wittkowski, J. and Moser, R. (2004) 'Psychological research on death attitudes: an overview and evaluation', *Death Studies*, vol 28, pp 309–40.

Neuberger, J. (2003) 'A healthy view of dying', *British Medical Journal*, vol 327, no 7408, pp 207–8.

Neuberger, J. (2006) *The Moral State We're In: A Manifesto for a 21st century society*, updated edition, London: Harper Perennial.

NFDA (2006) www.nfda.org/Funeral Service Trends (accessed 22 September 2006).

NHS (2006) *NHS End of Life Care Programme Progress Report March 2006*. www.endoflifecare.nhs.uk

Nocon, A. and Qureshi, H. (1996*) Outcomes of Community Care for Users and Carers: A Social services perspective*, Buckingham: Open University Press.

Noppe, I.C. and Noppe, L.D. (1999) 'Review of "Death and Spirituality"', *Death Studies*, vol 23, no 6, pp 569-76.

Nosowska, G. (2004) 'A delay they can ill afford: delays in obtaining Attendance Allowance for older, terminally ill cancer patients, and the role of health and social care professionals in reducing them', *Health and Social Care in the Community*, vol 12, no 4, pp 283–7.

Nouwen, H. (1972) *The Wounded Healer*, New York, NY: Doubleday and Co.

Nuyen, A. (2000) 'Levinas and the euthanasia debate', *Journal of Religious Ethics*, vol 28, no 1, pp 119–35.

Nyatanga, B. (2002) 'Culture, palliative care and multiculturalism', *International Journal of Palliative Nursing*, vol 8, no 5, pp 240–46.

Nyatanga, B. (2003) 'Guest editorial. Multidisciplinary team leadership', *International Journal of Palliative Nursing*, vol 9, no 7, p 276.

O'Connor, L. (2005) 'Dying smart', *Christianity Today* (August), pp 47–8.

Office of Fair Trading (2001) *Funerals. A report of the OFT inquiry into the funerals industry*, London: OFT.

Ogden, R. and Young, M. (1998) 'Euthanasia and assisted suicide: a survey of registered social workers in British Columbia', *British Journal of Social Work*, vol 28, no 2, pp 161-75.

Osterweis, M., Solomon, F. and Green, M. (1984) *Bereavement, Reactions, Consequences and Care*, Washington, DC: National Press.

Oswin, M. (1991) *Am I Allowed to Cry? A study of bereavement amongst people who have learning difficulties*, London: Souvenir Press.

Ovretveit, J. (1993) *Coordinating Community Care*, Buckingham: Open University Press.

Owens, A. and Randhawa, G. (2004) '"It's my culture; they're very different": providing community-based "culturally competent" palliative care for South Asian people in the UK', *Health and Social Care in the Community*, vol 12, no 5, pp 414–21.

Paley, J. (2007) 'Spirituality and secularization: Nursing and the sociology of religion', *Journal of Clinical Nursing* (Online Early Articles), doi: 10.1111/j.1365-2702.2006.01917.x.

Parker, M. (2004) 'Medicalizing meaning: demoralization syndrome and the desire to die', *Australian and New Zealand Journal of Psychiatry*, vol 38, pp 765–73.

Parkes, C.M. (1993) Bereavement as a psychosocial transition: processes of adaptation to change', in D. Dickenson and M. Johnson (eds) *Death, Dying and Bereavement*, London: Sage/Open University Press.

Parkes, C.M. (1996) *Bereavement: Studies of Grief in Adult Life* (3rd edn), London: Routledge.

Parkes, C.M. (2006) *Love and Loss: The roots of grief and its complications*, Hove: Routledge.

Parkes, C.M., Laungani, P. and Young, B. (eds) (1996) *Death and Bereavement Across Cultures*, London: Routledge.

Payne, S., Chan, A., Chau, R., Seymour, J. and Holloway, M. (2005) 'Chinese community views: promoting cultural competence in palliative care', *Journal of Palliative Care*, vol 21, no 2, pp 111–16.

Payne, S., Hillier, R., Langley-Evans, A. and Roberts, T. (1996) 'Impact of witnessing death on hospice patients', *Social Science and Medicine*, vol 43, no 12, pp 1785–94.

Payne, S., Seymour, J., Holloway, M. and Chapman, A. (2005) *Exploring and understanding the views of older Chinese people about cancer and end-of-life care*, Final Report to the Health Foundation (August).

Pearce, M., Singer, J. and Prigerson, H. (2006) 'Religious coping among caregivers of terminally ill cancer patients: main effects and psychosocial mediators', *Journal of Health Psychology*, vol 11, pp 743–59.

Pendergast, T. (2001) 'Advance care planning: pitfalls, progress, promise', *Critical Care Medicine*, vol 29, no 2, pp 34–9.

Peterson, M. (2000) 'A good death', *Christianity Today* (May) pp 64–9.

Pharos (1980) 'Non–religious funerals', *Pharos*, vol 46, pp 139–50.

Pharos International (2004) 'Disposition of cremated remains in Great Britain', *Pharos International*, 70, p 20.

Philpott, T. (ed) (1989) *Last Things: Social work with the dying and bereaved*, Birmingham: Community Care/Reed Publications.

Pickering, M., Littlewood, J. and Walter, T. (1997) 'Beauty and the beast: sex and death in the tabloid press', in D. Field, J. Hockey and N. Small (eds) *Death, Gender and Ethnicity*, London: Routledge, pp 124–41.

Pollack, C. (2003) 'Returning to a safe area? The importance of burial for return to Srebrenica', *Journal of Refugee Studies*, vol 16, no 2, pp 186-201.

Portenoy, R., Coyle, N., Ksh, K., Brescia, F., Scanlon, C. and O'Hare, D. (1997) 'Determinants of the willingness to endorse assisted suicide: a survey of physicians, nurses and social workers', *Psychosomatics*, vol 38, pp 277–87.

Priestly, M. (2000) 'Dropping 'E's: The missing link in quality assurance for disabled people', in A. Brechin, H. Brown and M. Eby (eds) *Critical Practice in Health and Social Care*, London: Sage/Open University Press.

Prigerson, H. and Jacobs, S. (2001) 'Diagnostic criteria for traumatic grief', in M. Stroebe, R. Hansson, W. Stroebe and H. Schut (eds) *Handbook of Bereavement Research: Consequences, coping and care*, Washington DC: American Psychological Association, pp 614–46.

Prigerson, H., Jacobs, S., Bradley, E. and Kasl, S. (2003) 'Letter. A good death is an oxymoron without consideration of mental health', *British Medical Journal*, vol 327, no 7408, pp 222.

Rahner, K. (1963) *On the Theology of Death*, New York, NY: Herder and Herder.

Rando, T. (1986) *Loss and Anticipatory Grief*, Lexington, MA: Lexington Books.

Raphael, B. (1992) *The Anatomy of Bereavement* (2nd edn), London: Hutchinson.

Rassool, G.H. (2004) 'Commentary: an Islamic perspective', *Journal of Advanced Nursing*, vol 46, no 3, pp 270–83.

Reb, A. (2003) 'Palliative and end-of-life care: policy analysis', *Oncology Nursing Forum*, vol 30, no 1, pp 35–50.

Reese, D. and Sontag, M.-A. (2001) 'Successful interprofessional collaboration on the hospice team', *Health and Social Work*, vol 26, no 3, pp 167–75.

Reimers, E. (1999) 'Death and identity: graves and funerals as cultural communication', *Mortality*, vol 4, no 2, pp 147–66.

Reisman, A. (2001) 'Death of a spouse: illusory basic assumptions and continuation of bonds', *Death Studies*, vol 25, pp 445–60.

Rentz, C., Krokorian, R. and Keys, M. (2004–5) 'Grief and mourning from the perspective of the person with the dementing illness: beginning the dialogue', *Omega*, vol 50, pp 165–79.

Roberts, P. (2004) 'Here today and cyberspace tomorrow: memorials and bereavement support on the web', *Generations*, vol 28, no 11, pp 41–6.

Robinson, S. (2002) '"Thanks for the memory ..." Death of a student: memorials, mourning and postmodernity', *Contact*, no 138, pp 16–25.

Ronel, N. and Lebel, U. (2006) 'When parents lay their children to rest: between anger and forgiveness', *Journal of Social and Personal Relationships*, vol 23, pp 507–22.

Rosenblatt, P. (1993) 'Grief: the social context of private feelings', in M. Stroebe, W. Stroebe and R. Hanssen (eds) *Handbook of Bereavement: Theory, research and intervention*, Cambridge: Cambridge University Press.

Ross, H. (2001) 'Islamic Tradition at The End of Life', *MEDSURG Nursing*, vol 10, no 2, pp 83-7.

Rowe, D. (1989) *The Construction of Life and Death*, London: Fontana.

Rowe, M. (2003) 'Grave changes. Scattering ashes in contemporary Japan', *Japanese Journal of Religious Studies*, vol 30, no 1–2, pp 85–118.

Rumbold, B. (1986) *Helplessness and Hope: Pastoral care in terminal illness*, London: SCM Press.

Rumbold, B. (2002) (ed) *Spirituality and Palliative Care: Social and pastoral perspectives*, Oxford: Oxford University Press.

Russ, A and Kaufman, S. (2005) 'Family perceptions of prognosis, silence and the "suddenness" of death', *Culture, Medicine and Psychiatry*, vol 29, pp 103–23.

Rutledge, D. (2003) 'Models of palliative care: moving beyond hospice', *ONS News*, vol 18, no 10, p 1, pp 4–5.

Salvatore, T. (1999–2001) 'Elder suicide primer: introduction to a late life tragedy', www.suicidereferencelibrary.com/ (accessed 6 November 2006).

Samaritans (1990) *Who Cares if I Live or Die? Suicide in Great Britain*, Slough: The Samaritans.

Sartre, J.-P. (1956) *Being and Nothingness*, ET New York, NY, Philosophical Library.

Saunders, C. (ed) (1990) *Hospice and Palliative Care: An Interdisciplinary Approach*, London: Edward Arnold.

Saysell, E. (2004) 'Pilot project of an intermediate palliative care unit within a registered care home', *International Journal of Palliative Nursing*, vol 10, no 8, pp 393–8.

Schiff, R., Rajkumar, C. and Bulpitt, C. (2000) 'Views of elderly people on living wills: interview study', *British Medical Journal*, vol 320, pp 1640–41.

Scrutton, S. (1995) *Bereavement and Grief: Supporting older people through loss*, London: Edward Arnold.

Seale, C. (1995a) 'Dying alone', *Sociology of Health and Illness*, vol 17, pp 377–91.

Seale, C. (1995b) 'Heroic death', *Sociology*, vol 29, pp 597–613.

Seale, C. (1998) *Constructing Death: The sociology of dying and bereavement*, Cambridge: Cambridge University Press.

Seale, C. (2000) 'Changing patterns of death and dying', *Social Science and Medicine*, vol 51, pp 917–30.

Seale, C. (2006) 'National survey of end-of-life decisions made by UK medical practitioners', *Palliative Medicine*, vol 20, pp 3–10.

Seale, C. and Cartwright, A. (1994) *The Year Before Death*, Aldershot: Avebury.

Searcey, D. (2006) 'On Iraq's front lines, digital memorials for fallen friends', *Wall Street Journal*, Eastern edition (26 January).

Seaton, J. (2006) 'The Old Black', *The Guardian*, 03.01.06, pp 24-5.

Seay, G. (2005) 'Euthanasia and physicians' moral duties', *Journal of Medicine and Philosophy*, vol 30, pp 517–33.

Seden, J. (1999) *Counselling Skills in Social Work Practice*, Buckingham: Open University Press.

Seymour, J. (2003) 'Technology and "natural death": a study of older people', *Zeitschrift fur Gerontologie und Geriatrie*, vol 36, no 5, pp 339–46.

Seymour, J.E., Witherspoon, R., Gott, M., Ross, H. and Payne, S. (2005) *End of Life Care: Promoting comfort, choice and well being among older people facing death*, Bristol: The Policy Press.

Seymour, J., Payne, S., Chapman, A. and Holloway, M. (2007) 'End of life care: expectations and experiences of white indigenous and Chinese older people in the UK', *Sociology of Health and Illness*, Monograph 13, 'Ethnicity, health and health care: understanding diversity, tackling disadvantage, vol 29, no 6 (DOI 10.1111/j.1467-9566.2007.01045.x)

Sheldon, F. (1997) *Psychosocial Palliative Care: Good practice in the care of the dying and bereaved*, Cheltenham: Stanley Thornes.

Sidell, M., Katz, J. and Komaromy, C. (1997) 'Death and dying in residential and nursing homes for older people: examining the case for palliative care.' Unpublished report, London: Department of Health.

Sieger, C., Arnold, J. and Ahronheim, J. (2002) 'Refusing artificial nutrition and hydration: does statutory law send the wrong message?', *Journal of the American Geriatrics Society*, vol 50, no 3, pp 544–50.

Silverman, P. (2004) *Widow to Widow: How the Bereaved Help One Another*, 2nd edn, New York: Brunner-Routledge.

Small, N. (1997) 'Death and difference', in D. Field, J. Hockey and N. Small (eds) *Death, Gender and Ethnicity*, London: Routledge.

Small, N. (2001) 'Theories of grief: a critical review', in J. Hockey, J. Katz and N. Small (eds) *Grief, Mourning and Death Ritual*, Buckingham, Open University Press, pp 19–48.

Smith, W. (2006) 'Organizing Death: Remembrance and Re-collection', *Organization*, vol 13, no 2, pp 225–44.

Smith-Stoner, M. (2005) 'End-of-life needs of patients who practice Tibetan Buddhism', *Journal of Hospice and Palliative Nursing*, vol 7, no 4, pp 228–33.

Snidle, H. (1996) 'Pastoral care of the dying and bereaved', in P. Badham and P. Ballard (eds) *Facing Death*, Cardiff: University of Wales Press.

Social Services Inspectorate (1997) *Better Management, Better Care. The Sixth Annual Report of the Chief Inspector of the Social Services Inspectorate 1996/7*, London: The Stationery Office.

Stearns, P. (2004) 'Review of "Gary Laderman, Rest in Peace: A cultural history of death and the funeral home in twentieth-century America"', *Journal of Social History*, vol 38, no 2, pp 541–43.

Steele, K., Ribbe, M., Ahronheim, J., Hendrick, H., Selwyn, P., Forman, W. and Keay, T. (1999) 'Incorporating education on palliative care into the long-term care setting', *Journal of the American Geriatrics Society*, vol 47, no 7, pp 904–7.

Stewart, K., Challis, D., Carpenter, I. and Dickenson, E. (1999) 'Assessment approaches for older people receiving social care: coverage and content', *International Journal of Geriatric Psychiatry*, vol 14, pp 147–56.

Stoddart, E. (2006) 'The cost of floral tributes', *Contact*, 149, pp 28–37.

Stroebe, M. (2001) 'Bereavement research and theory: retrospective and prospective', *American Behavioral Scientist*, vol 44, no 5, pp 854–65.

Stroebe, M. and Schut, H. (1999) 'The dual process model of coping with bereavement: rationale and description', *Death Studies*, vol 23, pp 197–224.

Stroebe, M. and Schut, H. (2005) 'To continue or relinquish bonds: a review of consequence for the bereaved', *Death Studies*, vol 29, pp 477–94.

Sudnow, D. (1967) *Passing On: The social organization of dying*, New York: Prentice Hall.

Tanner, D. (1998) 'Empowerment and care management: swimming against the tide', *Health and Social Care in the Community*, vol 6, no 6, pp 447–57.

Tarlow, S. (1999) *Bereavement and Commemoration. An Archaeology of Mortality*, London: Blackwell.

Taylor, B (2001) 'Views of nurses, patients and patients' families regarding palliative nursing care', *International Journal of Palliative Nursing*, vol 7, no 4, pp 186–91.

Tester, S. (1996) *Community Care for Older People: A Comparative Perspective*, Basingstoke: Macmillan.

Thomas, S. (2006) 'Parkinson's disease: a model for care', *Primary Health Care*, vol 16, no 8, p 18.

Thompson, N. (2002) 'Introduction', in N. Thompson (ed) *Loss and Grief: A guide for human services practitioners*, London: Palgrave, pp 1–20.

Thompson, S. (2002) 'Older people', in N. Thompson (ed) *Loss and Grief: A guide for human services practitioners*, London: Palgrave, pp 162–73.

Thursby, G. (1992) 'Islamic, Hindu and Buddhist conceptions of ageing', in T. Cole, D. van Tassel and R. Kastenbaum (eds) *Handbook of the Humanities and Aging*, New York, NY: Springer.

Tillich, P. (1959) 'The eternal now', in H. Feifel (ed) *The Meaning of Death*, New York, NY: McGraw-Hill.

Timmermans, S. (2005) 'Death brokering: constructing culturally appropriate deaths', *Sociology of Health and Illness*, vol 27, no 7, pp 993–1013.

Todd, C., Grande, G., Barclay, S. and Farquhar, M. (2002) 'General practitioners and district nurses views of hospital at home for palliative care', *Palliative Medicine*, vol 16, pp 251–4.

Townsend, J., Frank, A., Fermont, D., Dyer, S., Karran, O., Walgrove, A. and Piper, M. (1990) 'Terminal cancer care and patients' preferences for place of death: a prospective study', *British Medical Journal*, 301, pp 415–17.

Townsend, P. (1981) 'The structured dependency of the elderly: creation of social policy in the twentieth century', *Ageing and Society*, vol 1, pp 5–28.

Twomey, F., McDowell, D. and Corcoran, G. (Advance Access, 27 March 2007) 'End-of-life care for older patients dying in an acute general hospital – can we do better?', *Age and Ageing*.

Twycross, R. (1997) *Introducing Palliative Care*, 2nd edn, Abingdon: Radcliffe Medical Press.

Vandenthorpe, F. (2000) 'Funerals in Belgium: the hidden complexity of contemporary practices', *Mortality*, vol 5, no 1, pp 18–33.

Van Gennep, A. (1960) *The Rites of Passage*, London: Routledge and Kegan Paul.

Valverius, E., Nilstun, T. and Nilsson, B. (2000) 'Palliative care, assisted suicide and euthanasia: nationwide questionnaire to Swedish physicians', *Palliative Medicine*, vol 14, pp 141–8.

Verpoort, C., Gastmans, C., De Bal, N. and de Casterle, B. (2004) 'Nurses' attitudes to euthanasia: a review of the literature', *Nursing Ethics*, vol 11, no 4, pp 349–65.

Walker, A. (1981) 'Towards a political economy of old age', *Ageing and Society*, vol 1, pp 73–94.

Walker, A. and Maltby, T. (1997) *Ageing Europe*, Buckingham: Open University Press.

Walsh, K., King, M., Jones, L., Tookman, A. and Blizard, R. (2002) 'Spiritual beliefs may affect outcome of bereavement: prospective study', *British Medical Journal*, vol 324, pp 1551-54.

Walter, T. (1989) 'Secular funerals', *Theology*, vol 9, no 2, pp 394–402.

Walter, T. (1991) 'Modern death: taboo or not taboo?', *Sociology*, vol 25, no 2, pp 193–310.

Walter, T. (1993a) 'Death in the New Age', *Religion*, vol 23, pp 127–45.

Walter, T. (1993b) 'Sociologists never die: British sociology and death', in D. Clark (ed) *The Sociology of Death*, Oxford: Blackwell.

Walter, T. (1994) *The Revival of Death*, London: Routledge.

Walter, T. (1996) 'Funeral flowers: a Response to Drury', *Folklore*, vol 107, pp 106–7.

Walter, T. (1999) *On Bereavement: The culture of grief*, Buckingham: Open University Press.

Walter, T. (2003) 'Historical and cultural variants on the good death', *British Medical Journal*, vol 327, no 7408, pp 218–20.

Walter, T. (2004) 'Plastination for display: a new way to dispose of the dead', *The Journal of the Royal Anthropological Institute*, vol 10, no 3, pp 603–72.

Walter, T. (2005) 'Three ways to arrange a funeral. Mortuary variation in the modern West', *Mortality*, 10:3, 173–92.

Walter, T., Littlewood, J. and Pickering, M. (1995) 'Death in the News: the public invigilation of private emotion', *Sociology*, vol 29, pp 579–96.

Walters, G. (2004) 'Is there such a thing as a good death?', *Palliative Medicine*, vol 18, pp 404–8.

Wallerstein, C. (2006) 'Losing a dad', *The Guardian* (6 June).

Wallis, J. (2001) 'Continuing bonds. Relationships between the living and the dead within contemporary spiritualism', *Mortality*, vol 6, pp 127–45.

Ward, D. (2004) 'The friendlier way back to dust and ashes', *The Guardian* (8 March).

Watson, C. (1997) '"Born a lady, became a princess, died a saint": the reaction to the death of Diana, Princess of Wales', *Anthropology Today*, vol 13, no 6, pp 3–7.

Weiser, P. and Ochsmann, R. (2005) 'Coping with disenfranchised grief: a content analysis of bereavement rituals', Paper to the 27th Annual Conference of the Association for Death Education & Counseling, New Mexico.

Williams, R. (1990) *A Protestant Legacy. Attitudes to Death and Illness among Older Aberdonians*, Oxford: Clarendon Press.

Williams, S. (1996) 'The case against euthanasia', in P. Badham and P. Ballard (eds) *Facing Death: An Interdisciplinary Approach*, Cardiff: University of Wales Press, pp 117-129.

Wilkes, L. and White, K. (2005) 'The family and nurse in partnership: providing day–to-day care for rural cancer patients', *Australian Journal of Rural Health*, vol 13, pp 121–26.

Wilson, G. (2000) *Understanding Old Age: Critical and global perspectives*, London: Sage.

Woods, L., Craig, J. and Dereng, N. (2006) 'Transitioning to a hospice program', *Journal of Hospice and Palliative Nursing*, vol 8, no 2, pp 103–11.

Wouters, C. (2002) 'The quest for new rituals in dying and mourning: changes in the we–I balance', *Body and Society, vol 8, no* 1, pp 1–27.

World Health Organisation (2007) Definition of Palliative Care http://www.who.int/cancer/palliative/definition/en/

Worden, J.W. (1982) *Grief Counselling and Grief Therapy*, 1st edn, London and New York, NY: Tavistock Publications.

Worden, J.W. (2003) *Grief Counselling and Grief Therapy*, 3rd edn, London and New York, NY: Brunner-Routledge.

Wrapson, D. (1999) 'Parallel funeral services', *Age and Ageing*, 28, pp 501–2.

Young, M and Cullen, L. (1996) *A Good Death. Conversations with East Londoners*, London: Routledge.

Zanskas, S. and Coduti, W. (2006) 'Eugenics, Euthanasia, and Physician Assisted Suicide: An Overview for Rehabilitation Professionals', *Journal of Rehabilitation*, vol 72, no 1, pp 27-34.

Index

Page references for notes are followed by n

C

D

E

F

G

H

I

J

K

L

M

N

O

P

Q

R

V

W

Y

Z